# Aligned for Success

## Reset Your Body from the Ground Up

*How to Reach Your Fitness Goals,
Prevent Pain and Injury, and
Achieve Optimal Performance in
Work, Sports, and Life*

*Kitty —
Wishing you optimal health
for life !  Brenda Shaeffer PT, DPT*

## Dr. Brenda Shaeffer

City Point Press

Published by
City Point Press
(203) 571-0781
www.citypointpress.com

Distributed to the book trade by Simon & Schuster

Drawings © Heather Macintosh
Photographs © Kris Sullivan
Book and cover design by Barbara Aronica-Buck

ISBN: 978-1-947951-11-2
ebook ISBN: 978-1-947951-12-9

Manufactured in the United States of America

# Contents

# Foreword

As an amateur national and international Olympic athlete and coach, achieving and maintaining a high level of physical fitness is, and always has been, one of the most important parts of my life and career. Over time, I started to have pain in my back from years of training and competition, and it became severe enough to affect nearly all aspects of my life. Eventually, the pain shut me down. MRIs of my back verified why I had intractable pain and could no longer function at home or work, or even perform mundane daily tasks, such as driving, without pain and leg numbness.

At that point, I sought the expertise of Dr. Brenda Shaeffer, who evaluated, assessed, and realigned my body. She taught me how to maintain these changes and apply new ways to move in all parts of my life to protect my injured area. She figured out a blueprint to help me understand why my body hurt, how I was going to heal, be able to run again, and move forward. Although medications and injections temporarily reduced my severe pain, Dr. Shaeffer taught me the changes I needed to make to my physical alignment to stay active. She instantly improved how I understood my injuries, showed me how to listen to my body's cues and, as a result, I resumed all my activities, modifying them to match the realities of how to avoid further problems. In fact, I continue to lead my normal, physically active lifestyle. I have returned to running three to four times per week and using the elliptical and other machines the rest of the week. I am coaching, and remain very active in my three children's lives without pain as a regular presence. I have learned through Dr. Shaeffer how to translate the pain I feel on occasion, and what tools to use to stop it before it builds. My back MRI still shows the consequences of my very active life and athletic career, but I no longer have to be fearful of what this means for my future. I can move forward in my life.

In her new book *Aligned for Success: Reset Your Body from the Ground Up*, Dr. Shaeffer combines her years of experience, training, and education with the latest medical research to provide simple yet effective tools we all need to feel better, grow stronger, and help prevent pain or injuries. She reveals her scientifically sound method of "Thinking in Threes" and teaches us how to **rethink, recognize, and reset** our bodies. Dr. Shaeffer quickly and safely taught me the necessary changes I needed to make in my physical alignment, and how to maintain it to become pain free without any invasive surgeries!

I now have the confidence to continue with all the physical activities in my profession, as well as my daily health activities. I am forever grateful!

> – Carin Gabarra
> Head Soccer Coach, US Naval Academy
> 1991 US Soccer World Champion
> 1996 US Olympic Gold Medalist

# Preface

*Aligned for Success* is intended for anyone who is ready to stop and rethink how to use their body. Within this book you will recognize and apply new facts about your body, learn a few basic skills, and discover what tools to use and when to use them. You will regain confidence in making decisions about how to reach your optimal health and well-being. You will be able to take immediate action in resetting your body to move, rest, recover, and repair as it was designed to do. Learn how to make the next "right" decision, not just the "best," when solving your health issues.

*Aligned for Success* presents a predictive, proactive, and restorative system to eliminate the guesswork in finding that balance needed to restore your body's abilities. By learning and becoming confident in the three-step method: rethink, recognize, and reset, you will be able to make improvements at any age or stage of your life. Reset freedom of motion by fundamentally understanding natural movement and how your body is designed to support, transport, and restore itself. Take the right three steps in decision-making every time you have pain, an injury, or hit a performance plateau in sports or work. The three-step method is a tool which can help prevent and reduce the effects of the most preventable issues facing the healthcare community and population today. Learning how to use the three-step method helps a person become a skilled operator of their own body, and to attain, maintain, and control optimal performance in health and well-being for life.

# Introduction

In 1978, I had a front row seat at the birth of the fitness industry as it is interpreted in the United States today. In December of that year, as a new physical therapist, I attended the first research educational fitness conference, where scientists corroborated new evidence to develop guidelines for adults to move and stay healthy. America had become increasingly sedentary and mechanized, with more cars, less community, more processed foods, and with the busied lifestyle in full swing. Physical therapists had been becoming more involved with the concepts of whole-body health, not just joint range of motion, modalities, and/or strengthening as a remedy. We began integrating fitness into our therapies, but no real guidelines for proper mechanics or safety had been concretely established. During the conference, I had the pleasure to talk with Jesse Owens, who was also the keynote speaker, in a room full of enthusiastic physical therapists, exercise scientists, and physicians, all interested in trying to make determinations on how to keep American adults physically fit. Mr. Owens's thoughts on this topic (after he put out his cigarette in an ashtray at the speaker's podium) were that we should remember to be respectful to our bodies; we should listen to our bodies and realize that by the time we are forty-five years old, we have lived half our lives, and that we should be grateful for that, and realize our abilities will naturally decline and we must alter our expectations to match this reality. In addition, he felt that injury prevention and determining fitness guidelines would not be needed if we applied common health practices: eating well, exercising, resting, and finding the balance within all applications. This was also the advice in the formative years for fundamental exercise rules which was published in a primer for primary though college-aged students in 1884 (Smith, 1884 [See pages 156–158 for full citations]). We did not listen to the advice of Mr. Owens or the wise observances of the physicians from nearly one hundred years prior. At the time of the conference, the fitness industry was focused on cardio because of the sedentary lifestyles that abounded. Weight loss was the primary goal in fitness programs. After that conference, the development of fitness and intentional "health" concepts and the consequences we are now living with today included high-impact aerobics, lots of reps with muscle work based largely on the single muscle-building model from earlier fitness muscle competitions, stretching, which was thought to be good if you had pain to "lengthen" the muscles, and dramatic changes in food source engineering and processing. This approach, over the next fifteen years, led to a rapidly increasing rate of overuse syndromes from too much joint impact without adequate rest or recovery, massive numbers of osteoarthritis (wear and tear on joints loaded incorrectly over and over), obesity levels never before seen, and pain needs "managed" with drugs at an epidemic level.

To put it plainly, I also did not find the balance I needed. I had a large outpatient orthopedic physical therapy practice I owned with another PT with five different locations at one point, and had gotten caught up in the insurance-driven game of PT, dictated by the numbers. Quantity not quality became the force and reality, even when it was not the intent. Research was beginning to become clearer in how the body works, especially with the most common issues—pain in the low back, neck, knee, and shoulder not caused by an accident or obvious incident—I would see in the orthopedic setting. Physical therapy at that time was outdated, and included performing exercises in a specific area where pain presented itself, providing manual therapy, stretching everything and strengthening the "core," hoping the patient would just reach their goals. But that approach was missing key elements. The words "closed chain," "kinetic chain," and "functional" were very new age at that point. I continued to strive to keep up with the research and apply the findings to my patients' issues. "Spine stabilization" and "core" became very popular in the 1980s but continued to focus on the mid-abdomen and largely ignore the whole body, while Pilates and yoga were becoming more popular across the country. Something was missing. Connecting the gym and exercise "class" model to real life and natural movements, and properly loading the body was fundamentally missing. I let myself become a victim of my own profession, and previous injuries caught up with me. A turning point for me came in 2005, when the newest and most definitive research on the brain regarding pain and biomechanics was becoming clearer. That information came at a time I personally needed it the most. In about 1972, I had been training as a highly competitive gymnast, and during a meet fell onto my bent neck from about nine feet high when I missed catching the high bar. I landed on a concrete floor covered by a canvas cotton batting mat, injuring my spine at two levels, eventually creating a forty-five-degree scoliosis over the years from poor treatment.

By 2005, I was having difficulty using my left leg reliably on stairs. My leg would often give way, a numbness developed in it, and a large shift of the vertebra had occurred with the instability. The new findings of biomechanists in those years confirmed this and put the injury result in perspective; T2 and T3 plus L1 and L2 (thoracic and lumbar combined) only have six millimeters (less than half an inch). Therefore, there was much more of the spine intact than broken. Even so, three out of three surgeons insisted I needed a four-to-six level fusion with very high risks involved and a long recovery. And there would be serious doubts about my ability to continue practicing physical therapy. I was a competitive sailboat racer at that time, but that also would likely stop. The reality that my life was about to change completely was settling in. A new normal was now saying "no" more often than "yes" to the very activities that I loved to do. Inactivity reinforced the path that led to the systematic self-imposed limitations. Stretching and performing "strength" exercises had replaced living my life's goals. The pain I felt as a physical therapist unable to fix my own issues was crushing me. My former PT partners intervened, telling me I was being irresponsible for not having surgery.

However, something from my past gymnastics and dance training, as well as my inherited common sense (Dad's mechanical engineer brain) kept playing in my head. Reflecting on my past experience and success in gymnastics reminded me that successful performance had always come due to hard work and lots of practice. But the method was practicing the part of a "trick" (or move) or combination of moves that I could not perform. We did not perform movements unless they included a component that we were going to perform in our routines. The lesson learned was that *relevant training*, i.e., matching the task involved with the goal, was essential. The solution was still not obvious because of the gold standard medical/PT approaches of the time. So, I consulted a physical therapy associate, Richard Jackson, a brilliant therapist who introduced me to Stuart McGill, PhD, spine biomechanist at Waterloo University of Ontario, Canada. Working with him and understanding the findings developed from his research and applications relevant to my issues became the beginnings of the solution. I went back to the basics from my gymnastics past. That combined with the confidence gained from finally having the research data support what I had experienced, gave me the skills I needed to apply to my own body. With this new perspective, new research, and applying the lessons learned from new science, I carefully began to rebuild and reset my body's abilities from the feet up, eventually reaching my goal of returning to work and life pain-free most of the time, without any medications or surgery. Within four months, I was back to most activities and also returned to sailing, both offshore and in dinghies, competitively. In fact, in 2008 I completed the Avon Walk, which consisted of a marathon distance the first day and a half-marathon distance the second, sleeping on the ground in a tent between the two, all with no pain. My focus shifted from what I couldn't do to what I could do, and how to understand my capabilities with confidence.

Too often, due to lack of knowledge and unclear current research-based approaches to solve issues, there is an unnecessary level of disability self-imposed by patients. Sadly, our most common perceptions of what is true has created a disabled "cannot" population versus an able "can" population.

I can now perform all types of daily, sport, and work-related activities within the context of my diagnosis, not defined by my diagnosis. I have learned how to read the language of my pain and other symptoms in my body, thereby modifying my training and making sure the alignment of my joints is maintained throughout movement sequences and supported when still from the feet up. I have learned to increase my abilities with what I was able to do without increasing my symptoms. This became the new plan of action instead of focusing on "fixing" the two segments of my back. I learned that even with a large diagnosis, a systematic method of implementing strategies that work around (not ignore) the diagnosis, combined with rest and natural movement sequences, facilitates successful healing, and allows patients to accomplish goals, take control, and have the freedom to live life.

Gymnastics training and my injuries propelled me to question the standards that largely focused on body-building-based movements to remedy the issues most common within orthopedics, sports injury prevention, and work performance.

This approach had emerged in the 1980s and continues to be a prevalent approach today. Body building as a competitive activity for aesthetics and sport is composed of singular muscle strength for bulk building. However, natural human movement patterns are generally in diagonal patterns, and result from a relatively rapid sequence of loading and unloading joints with muscles that are contracting and relaxing to control the angle of motion and speed. This creates the force necessary for tasks to be completed, while balancing the body as a whole to stay upright. Research has determined that best results for restoring or improving natural movement come from performing an activity repeatedly by mimicking the same environment: speed, forces (with optimal loading at joints), range of motion, and endurance of an activity. Dr. McGill teaches that there is a missed training opportunity when one is not mimicking the relevant activity. The goal is to eliminate the "energy leaks" caused by poor joint alignment, which creates less than optimal loading and unloading of the joints, and forces the brain to find a default, alternate movement sequence to stay upright. Loading the skeleton (structure) in the most appropriate sequence allows the skeletal parts and tissues attached to them to support, be recruited, and used most efficiently. This ability of our brain to instantly and repeatedly adjust our alignment and muscle use at a precise time is a great advantage for survival and the body's adaptation process. Although the process of adaptation is an awesome survival process, it is not sustainable, because there is an imbalance of resources used and eventually, the body parts will break down. This results in a lack of circulation from compression at the joints in addition to abnormal muscle forces changing mechanical advantages, resulting in less than optimal strength, balance, and range of motion.

My experiences inspired me to rethink the way to assess and teach patients about their own bodies' performance and how to recover optimal potential. The first step in reaching your goals is to expediently identify the exact cause of the issue hindering you (Duthey, 2013).

That does not mean an L5 bulge is the issue at hand. The issue may actually pertain to the surrounding parts of the body that have caused the L5 to bulge. Once you have determined the problem, you need to create a measurable goal. Without a goal, you cannot gauge progress. And who is helping you attain this goal? As a consumer, you should know every one of your solution team member's credentials.

Finally, to reach your goal, implementing an action plan to reset to your optimal ability may take time, but with practice and patience, and following the three-step method, you will begin to see results.

I learned that the human body moves in predictable, repeatable patterns. Confidence returning from my own success in recovering from my injury, coupled with the new evidence and knowledge of how training optimal performance should be done, drastically changed my perspective regarding injury, performance assessment, and solution strategies. I also began reminding patients to alter their expectations for successful goal attainment. The additional missing element was educating people on how to properly utilize tools, or perform activities guided by the cues from listening to and understanding their body's language. The knowledge learned from brain and biomechanics research gave me the basis for the clinical application to develop a practical approach anyone can use to get immediate results in improved health and performance. Thus, the concepts behind *Aligned for Success* were born.

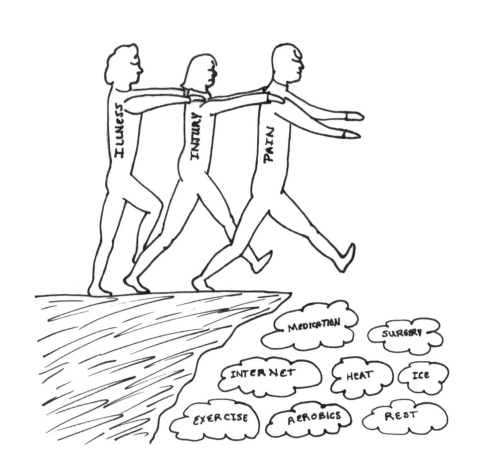

# What We Thought versus What We Now Know

## New Facts

The method outlined in this book will help you reset your body from the ground up, based on the latest in biomechanics combined with your body's natural tendencies. The three-step method (*rethink, recognize, reset*) is based also on common sense, but there are many reasons that this has not been developed before. Let's face it, "quagmire" is the only word to describe the current pathway to the right—not necessarily the best—health decision-making. We are in a prevalent state of confusion and indecisive approaches, which very often result in re-injuries. There is a lot of scientific evidence and user-friendly information available to attain and maintain the best health for ourselves. However, self-care management attempts often lead to unnecessary, late, or wrong diagnoses. The internet genesis has convoluted the medical decision-making process by showcasing what is popular rather than what is supported and proven scientific data. Beliefs prevail that a shoe, an exercise, a pill, a vitamin, surgery, or just plain hope will cure the issue.

Our culture relies on WikiHow to tell us when, what, and how to do activities, simply forgetting that these sources, although readily available, are not always reliable or from qualified, up-to-date medical professionals. We seem to have lost both our common sense and our self-reliance, because we now do not have to think or learn for ourselves—we can simply Google it. With all of the available resources, we still are lacking a road map for the most basic preventable human issues and maintenance of body breakdowns and pain. The time has come to adopt a method based in reality, one that's scientifically proven. We humans are surprisingly resilient, self-healing, and empowered beings. Our healing starts first with rethinking what we have adopted to be true and reentering with an open mind to develop a plan to reach our goals. To move forward, it is essential for you to review and recognize new facts, and to understand how these facts demand new thinking that could change your plan for success. We need to make sure we are operating in reality. Previous research, without the benefit of technology, led to teaching countless aerobic dancers how to "pelvic tilt"—only later was it discovered that such a move promoted disc problems (McGill, 1998).

We thought isolating a single muscle group had relevance to natural movement. We thought that the strength of single muscle groups could only be measured by a machine, disregarding range of motion, speed, and force as viable measurements. Core exercises were introduced to help reduce back pain (McGill, 1998). Touching your toes to stretch your hamstrings without regards to keeping the curve in your back was overlooked, and created unstable lower backs and disc injuries (Mcgill,1998). Fortunately, we are learning from our past mistakes through research and the benefits of now having advanced technology. Some of the new information can be somewhat alarming because there have been recent changes that are not consistent with popular beliefs and practices used today. I have picked my favorite facts (below) that I refer to daily in my own research and practice. As the world of technology meets the world of movement and brain science, we can all benefit from well-researched findings. Interestingly, these findings date back to 1840s theories about body mechanics that were written in early primers of health and physiology in the United States when there was a need to define health and wellness practices. Common sense and practicality is the rule of thumb. Learning these facts, and understanding the resulting benefits, have helped my patients move forward in reaching their goals.

Following are the basic facts concerning the body's structures and causes of pain and performance failures, and then the benefits to implementing the program by resetting your body.

**Fact:** Feet contain twenty-six bones and are the first responders to pressure of our body every time we get up to move. They are the first shock absorbers (mini trampolines) necessary for best body support and movement.

**Benefit:** Your feet are the body's first and last base of support. They promote circulation and initialize movement for your whole body. An incorrect base will create a chain reaction of issues and problems from the feet up. Starting from the ground up will rebalance and reset your whole body.

**Fact:** Eighty-five to ninety-five percent of muscular-skeletal pain or performance issues are from non-specific and multi-factorial causes. In other words, not from one trauma or disease. (Duthey, 2013)

**Benefit:** Most issues are progressive or happen "off the field," a result of a person not necessarily paying close attention to their bodies when they are working out, exercising, or training. A consequence of this is less-than-optimal alignment during the more mundane, automatic movements, such as slouching, washing dishes, walking/running, picking up groceries, driving, carrying one child on one hip, looking down while texting, etc. In turn, the brain and body have to adapt to these movements and breakdown ensues after inadequate recovery, circulation, support, and repair time. This program will help you look at your body as a whole and avoid the most preventable injuries, pain, and performance issues.

**Fact:** The tight feeling is usually the result of muscles being forced to adapt from inappropriate movement or positioning on the opposite side of the body and/or a segment above or below them. The muscles are not weak; in fact, just the opposite. They are being overused or not allowed to relax or recover. That is why a muscle relaxed by techniques such as myofascial release, massage, or foam rolling often reverts to its previous tight feeling. Generally, this muscle is helping to balance your body in adjusting for a deficit in another area, which is usually on the opposite side of the same joint or body segment where you are experiencing the tight feeling. Newton's

Third Law of Physics—for every action there is an equal and opposite reaction—comes into play, because our bodies have to stay upright as we move through our tasks of the day. If you are only squatting and sitting all day and also sit predominantly on one of your pelvis bones, the thighs become imbalanced, using quadriceps more than hamstrings, causing a need to adjust muscular use from optimal to ensure you do not lose your balance as you sit, stand, or walk. The most common complaint seen over and over is the tight "IT band" or tight hamstring. This tightness is a signal from your brain telling you that these muscles have adapted so long and consistently to an imbalance in your posture, and is sounding an alarm for you to recognize there is an unsustainable situation. Toxins have built to a level that there is no time or opportunity to remove them, causing an unsustainable muscle/tendon action that creates a sensation of tightness in the outside quadriceps. The hamstring, having been silenced all day, is actually underutilized. It is needed but not ready for action, so when called to action, it contracts quickly, therefore giving the warning signal of tightness. This most often is seen in the presence of overstretched hamstrings plus over-strengthened quadriceps ("quad" dominance or imbalanced strength) combined with lack of hip control, especially gluteal group, and chronic slouching or excessive core forward bending. The other most common complaint is that the "traps," the muscles in the upper middle back, are tight and the cause given is stress. The reality is that inadequate natural recruitment and use of the latissimus dorsi ("lats"), arm support, alignment of the head over the shoulders, rest and recovery, leave the traps no choice by the brain but to be used to literally keep the head from falling forward, and keep the arms and shoulders from falling down the ribcage. Also, tightness has been a documented result of fear.

**Benefit:** Alignment correction is the first and most important step to take to reset your body for optimal use. Learning the language of your body, and becoming skilled in knowing how to attain then maintain appropriate alignment, provides balance of musculature and support, and will allow recovery and appropriate readiness for daily activities. Recognizing the adaptations your brain has been making over time, then systematically correcting the alignment, first allows the expected results from the strength and stretching applied in the correct order with alignment. Tightness and pain restriction when there is chronic pain could be because the subconscious brain is very strong, and education must be the first approach, proven to increase mobility, rather than focusing on whether or not to stretch.

**Fact:** Fear about more pain, whatever the injury or issue actually is, decreases mobility and causes even more pain. Compounded issues related to loss of income, future plans related to unknowns of what the injury might mean, frustration, embarrassment, and disappointment from failed treatments, self-worth issues—all are proven to cause more fear, pain, and failure of treatments.

**Benefit:** Learning what pain is, how it can be controlled, and where it comes from with a musculoskeletal problem is proven to immediately increase mobility significantly (*Clinical Journal of Pain*). Educating the person having the pain issue using lay terms and specific real-life situations will optimize and accelerate goal attainment.

**Fact:** Tissues will heal if you give them the correct environment (ingredients) with intention (McGill, 2015).

**Benefit:** Learning the language of your body and taking time to heal with the correct tools will eliminate the fear that you will never get better. Recover, rest, and repair allows the body to regenerate and become ready for the next thing you choose to do.

**Fact:** Our brains can change (neuroplasticity) (McGill, 2015).

**Benefit:** With time, precision, and practice we can *reset* our bodies to optimal levels of performance. Neuromuscular re-training helps the brain develop new pathways so we don't have to default into our previous protective muscle sequence that had resulted in breakdown or less-than-optimal performance.

**Fact:** Opioids reduce the sensation of pain by interrupting pain signals to the brain.

**Benefit:** Opioids are a Band-Aid approach to the real issue, and may only prolong the problem. Kimberly Johnson,

PhD, director of the Center for Substance Abuse Treatment at the Substance Abuse and Mental Health Services Administration, says, "Avoid opioids if you are being treated for chronic pain. Physical therapy is more effective for long-term conditions like lower back pain and headache" (Johnson, 2017).

**Fact:** For adults less than fifty years old, without signs and symptoms of systemic disease (Parkinson's, multiple sclerosis, lupus, rheumatoid arthritis), diagnostic imaging (MRI, CT scan) does not improve the treatment outcome of low back pain (Duthey, 2013).

**Benefit:** Diagnostic imaging shows a snapshot, but does not show how the affected area is responding to different movements. Therefore, you can save both money and time by following the method in this book to help change structural alignment.

**Fact:** You have to look at and evaluate (*rethink*) the effectiveness of previous approaches and attempts in order to plan and finally reach your goals (Greene, Appel, Reinert, Palumbo, 2005).

**Benefit:** By rethinking previously failed results you can develop a problem-solving strategy. You have to have a plan based on accurate diagnosis, effective solution team members, and understanding of the benefits of previous treatments. Without this step, you are destined to repeat the same mistakes, waste time and money, and potentially cause more harm.

**Fact:** Your subconscious brain does not recognize "why" versus "how" you are using your body, and must help you be your best by adapting as necessary during all activities of your daily life.

**Benefit:** With recognition and intentional appropriate alignment maintained in all activities—not just the obvious activities, such as exercise class, but also the routine tasks of life—you must assess, correct, and consistently improve alignment to reset and use your body optimally for life.

**Fact:** When attempting to return to activity after injury, the first step is to return to cardio movement if pain needs to be controlled. More than ten minutes of movement, sustained with a heart rate of more than 50 percent of vo2max (the maximum amount of oxygen you use during an intense workout), will have a pain-reducing effect.

**Benefit:** Appropriate alignment is what makes structure strong and provides open space to get the toxins out and nutrients into the body tissues to allow healing. In addition, if a person increases their heart rate an average of twenty beats per minute, and maintains this for around forty-five minutes, their brain can produce 10 milligrams of a morphine-like chemical in the body to relieve pain. This can be done without impact if needed (Louw, Flynn, & Puentedura, 2015).

**Fact:** Ice should be used for short sessions when there has been an obvious injury, where there has been a break of tissues, or if the pain is intolerable. Otherwise, heat is always the first thing used for pain and should be used for ten-minute sessions frequently throughout the day, especially before bed.

**Benefit:** Heating helps improve circulation to the area, brings more fluids and removes toxins that have accumulated, and allows the joints and tissues to move more freely and relax. Think about how stiff you feel when you go out into the cold and how slowly you move. You are trying to restore movement and movement is rapid and fluid, not slow and stiff. The rules have changed. Make sure you understand when and why you are using heat and cold. Cold is sometimes used as a jump-start shock to flush out the waste in the body, but make sure the provider of the service is a licensed medical professional prepared for any body reaction if you have medical issues.

**Fact:** You must train to perform any activity within the same range of motion, speed, force, and movement pattern to improve within that specific activity. For example, if you are training for a 5K walk, yoga alone will not prepare you for that activity because it does not follow any of the criteria.

**Benefit:** Save time by not wasting money on exercise programs that do not match the positions, range of motion, speed, or force you are trying to correct or train to perform. To train for walking, reset your ability to balance, restore your feet, legs, arms, and core range of motion and strength to match the tasks of walking. Yoga is fantastic for brain focus, mediation, joint balance, breathing, and joint support, among other things. Prioritize your time and money to reset your body for your goals. For example, running already includes landing and pushing off the forefoot, so toe raises in a fitness program may create an overuse situation, since those muscles have already been worked. If bike racing is your sport, then you need to pay specific attention to the timing of how and when to counter-strengthen the muscles that hold you upright, as opposed to yoga or other stretches that may be more appropriate for front muscles of the body. On a bike, the front muscles are used excessively in controlling the bike. Remember that the muscles, heart, and organs of the body do not have eyes. They need balance and counterbalance, with rest and recovery included.

**Fact:** Core strengthening alone does not prevent back pain. Correcting sequence and balance of muscle use creates structural strength.

**Benefit:** Neuromuscular retraining is necessary for maintaining appropriate alignment in all aspects of life. Easy skill practices and exercises are used to reset then restore goal activity. By intentionally using your brain and structure to help train alignment patterns, you will create better support and strength.

**Fact:** Unless a violent injury has occurred, back joints, including the sacrum, do not go "out," but create pain resulting from inappropriate use and/or pressure on the joint and other structures, which decreases circulation creating congestion from strained and compressed tissues. The pain alarm signals from the brain occur when there is imminent damage to the systems of the body.

**Benefit:** General attention to recognize how you have been moving or maintaining a position, then resetting, along with heating for ten minutes to help improve circulation to the area, bring more fluids, remove toxins that have accumulated, and allows more nutrients to the compressed area to relieve the strain pattern. End result: savings of time and money.

## Learn the Language of the Body

To determine what is causing your most pressing issue, try not to use medical terms, but instead use your own words. Using medical language has been shown to create fear and sometimes paralyze decision-making (Vlaeyen & Linton, 2000). Fear can create anxiety and/or pain, wasting time and money, and leading to failure. Not to mention learning the medical terms for a diagnosis can become a crutch. For example, if someone has a bulging disc at L5, it can become a label that's difficult to discard. Fear predicts pain, often leading to a cycle difficult to break (George, Bialosky, Fritz, 2004). The reality is that only a small percentage of people with an L5 bulging disc attain their pain from the findings on an MRI (Duthey, 2013). The findings are more often than not resulting from adapted movement patterns your brain signals muscles to perform repeatedly to compensate for things such as slouching or injury. The pain and tightness sensation are often from sore muscles and a buildup of toxins from overuse or deterioration of bone endings from poor loading angles. One test result without careful assessment shouldn't dictate all future activities. Time lost with inappropriate treatments can lead to maladaptive brain neu-ropathways, which makes recovery less likely to occur. Old, out-of-date words can create a misunderstanding of key con-cepts, making health and performance solution decisions more difficult. These words provide the basis for fresh marketing spins promoting the fitness and health industry. Think of all the popular group activity fitness trends today that combine the science of exercise and health facts with sometimes unsub-stantiated claims. Obviously, best intentions and fancy mar-keting are designed to capture your attention and dollars. As with any service you buy, beware!

All of the latest fitness trends urge you to move, but each of them has its own unique niche marketing spin to engage consumers. Some examples of these words or phrases that are used to draw customers include: myofascial, heart-rate based interval training, isometric training, low-impact, high-intensity interval training (HIIT), suggesting an elevated importance or exclusivity of the services being advertised. Unfortunately, a lot of these places keep my physical therapy practice in busi-ness. Believing the providers of the program know your needs is dangerous and often not true. Confirm the credentials and intent of the programs you are enrolled in and how you can safely participate. Trusted, scientific evidence should never be replaced by anecdotal success or personal stories. People are often performing exercises using improper alignment and can end up prolonging their issues in the name of "exercise and health." For example, in the chiropractic and physical therapy world, joint positions are described as "out" or "subluxed," which leaves patients with the impression that realignment is necessary to "put them back" in, leading to further dependency on health professionals. Other buzz words are frequently attached to old information, creating fear, dependency, and hampering of progress through misleading objectives. Understanding the implications of new lessons learned from research, I suggest changing the use of certain terms and practice saying them in your daily life to promote a consistent language across all medical professions and health providers.

The language of your body is best understood when you work with professionals who use figures and measurements representative and specific for you. The focus of discussion must be relevant and include analysis in plain language of what has been tried, and why these approaches did or did not work for you. Many people slow down and/or stop progressing because they compare themselves to other people, either in a class or in photos or handouts. Dr. Admundson (Vlaeyen, Linton, 2000) found this tendency decreases potential for success, when patients simply cannot connect to what the medical professionals or health providers are trying to say. Consider the most common experience I have with patients after we've set up a plan to progress. Patients will go out of town, receive a massage treatment, go to a new exercise class, and the practitioner or class leader makes a comment such as "You have the tightest IT band I've ever seen!" or "Your rib is out" or "You have a leg length discrepancy." The usual response by the patient is immediate alarm, discouragement, fear, anxiety, and loss of confidence in the plan they had implemented with me to reach their goals.

This undermines the intention of the service/class the patient is participating in and can be an overwhelming surge of information. Take care to stay realistic and verify the definition of off-hand comments that a trainer, massage therapist, chiropractor, or physical therapist may say related to your actual issues. Such comments could lead to catastrophe and cause you to adapt to unnecessary movement restrictions or pain.

> **Patient Story:** *Mrs. H had come to me as a very timid exerciser about seven years ago, but still a very active healthcare participant, meaning she was going to three to five healthcare providers for various treatments weekly. She had been diagnosed with a multitude of both systemic issues, including allergy issues, and connective tissue problems, leading her to believe she was extremely fragile. She regularly turned down opportunities to go on family vacations and social events, and experienced frustration and fatigue. When I met her, we went over her history— her list of documented diagnoses, the healthcare providers and approaches of care she had received, and her response to these diagnoses. She always had a long list of medical words to ask me about, and suffered from fear caused by the use of these words that had been used by her providers to try to "educate" her. What we discovered was that several treatments were redundant, several more were admittedly not helpful, and another she reported actually caused pain, but she was too polite to let the professional know this. Hundreds of dollars and hours each*

*week were being spent, and there were no clear, measurable goals established. After careful assessment and a few visits to sort out her potential and development, she was advanced to a plan of learning the three-step method of* rethink, recognize, reset, *and with the help of a collaborating personal trainer and her personal physician, the number of visits to all health-related persons decreased to three to four visits per month. Within a year, she was participating again in social and family events and has been able to maintain an optimal level of health related to her medical issues. She now admits that she regularly reminds and instructs others in corrective alignment skills she has learned to help her manage her present medical conditions.*

As you learn how to recognize, react to your body, and "read" the language of your body, you will then understand the resetting corrections to make to produce the expected results. Understanding the language of your body bridges the gap between society and medical health professionals and allows you to understand the medical lingo involved in your particular condition and how it relates to the issue you are attempting to address. Simply learning this information has been proven to keep the brain as calm as possible and allow best outcomes (Louw, Diener, & Puentedura, 2014). This ultimately leads to you being the best resource tool to be able to make accurate decisions for your health without requiring instruction or learning a "foreign" language. Our body structure can be adjusted for, and tolerate, rather large differences in ranges of motions and muscle lengths by the brain and still survive. It is designed for that. Your brain can make the relatively minor adjustments to still have efficient, effective, and safe movement. In a year of patients, I usually have only one or two with actual bone length differences, as opposed to differences in the length of the leg resulting from adapting for an injury or pain. Understand that unless there is a big leg length difference (i.e., can be seen from across a room) due to bones actually being a different length, there is no rationale to implement modifications. This includes depending immediately on orthotics for "flat feet" without working on alignment first. Do not be caught up in the hype and focus on the possibility of leg length differences and the flat feet pitch. Also, be wary of a quick diagnosis and assumptions of decreased potential for performance secondary to these claims. Your body is an amazing gift, designed to move, adjust, repair, recover, and work for your lifetime. After you learn how to reset your body and understand the language of your body, you will enjoy a more pain-free and confident life of "can do."

# Body Basics:
# The Three Systems of the Body

## Structure: The Container, Form, and Mover

Before we can fully dive into the three-step method, an understanding of simple body basics is essential. Please complete the Geography of Your Structure Worksheet on page 121 to find and learn the geographical landmarks of your skeletal structure that will be necessary in order to apply the method taught in this book. The body is designed to operate simultaneously within three systems. They are all interrelated and dependent upon each other: the structural system, the fluid/nutrition system, and the nervous system, which includes the brain, spinal cord, and nerves. The anatomy of the body describes how all the individual parts of the body are joined together. The physiology describes how all systems interact and work together. You will need an accurate understanding of each system and what they are designed to do. With this knowledge you will be able to recognize your own needs within the context of the three systems at work. Your body is a wonderful gift. It is not a machine, but a regenerative, resilient organism when maintained and managed appropriately. Taking care of your body is a choice. This is not a practice run, but the only opportunity we have to make the right decisions and actions with the bodies we are given. Keeping solutions as simple as possible will allow you to rapidly learn the skills and tools you need to help you reach your goals with confidence and competence, regardless of the bombardment of information about how to accomplish this over the years. Remember that a healthy body is not just a goal but a continuous state of being.

**Patient Story:** *Kendall Tant—Kendall was a very active guy in his fifties. He exercised vigorously three to four times per week, primarily biking, mountain biking, and bike riding on the beach. The issue he was having when he first came to see me was general muscle tightness and knee pain that he could not resolve. We assessed the position of his body on his bike and found that he was not aligned for successful joint loading. He learned how his muscles, tendons, and skeleton all affect each other, and we taught him stretches pertaining to his particular issues. With the help of some dry needling (see Glossary on p. 159) he was able to find relief. He still remains as active as ever, but the knee pain and muscle tightness he was experiencing are completely gone.*

The structure system supports, provides form, and moves the entire body and serves as a container for the components of the nervous and nutrient/fluid systems. The structure also includes the containers for vital organs such as the heart, lungs, stomach, blood and lymph vessels, and nerves with surrounding fascia, and holds everything in place. Structure is your shape, and how you are recognized by others. The structure is also the skeleton, muscles, and all tissues, including joint-connecting ligaments, capsules and all connective tissue (fascia) that wraps around and provides support for all organs and tissues. Without fascia, your biceps would fall from the front of your arm to the bottom as you move, and there would be no way to contain lubricating muscles. The primary challenge for your structure is supporting you as you either stay in a position for an extended period of time or move at rapid speeds over a period of time in any direction, i.e., pushing, pulling, and/or lifting. The body has to react to gravity to stay upright while still completing tasks, unless you are fully supported and parallel to gravity and ground. You inherit the shape, dimensions, and sturdiness of the materials, which include capabilities and performance potential. Some people have very flexible connective tissue, which does not respond well to high-impact activities, whereas others have stiffer tissue and naturally have a spring-like response to high impact, and survive better over time in those types of activities. Some people are given connective tissue and other structure building blocks made of heavy-duty materials; others are more fragile—corduroy versus silk. Thick-boned versus slightly built bones predict the performance capabilities for the structure when a task in an activity is performed. Recognizing your history and performance capabilities and developing goals and plans appropriate for these realities will result in less injury risk and optimal results.

**Patient Story:** *Jill Monroe Schumacher, PA—Jill has been a patient with me for over seven years. She wasn't an athlete growing up, but she was a gymnast for a couple of years and sustained her fair share of injuries. Since then has moved on from that sport. She picked up running when she was twenty-eight years old. She remembers it being very difficult at the beginning. She felt like she had an injury every couple of months. She finally called a local running store and said: "Tell me the best physical therapist in town! I don't care where I go or how much it will cost." Like many people, she was tired of having so many repetitive injuries. To this day, I still see Jill and we were able to get to the bottom of her issue. We were able to correct posture issues, including how to sit at work, drive in her car (I even suggested car pedal extensions for her petite body), sit at home, and run. Because Jill is a physician's assistant, she understands how the body works. We just used that to her advantage so she could apply simple tools to help her with proper alignment. She uses little cues I've given her along the way to make minor adjustments that helped with major improvements in her running. One example is her foot placement while she was running. Jill was unaware of how she landed and the placement of her foot, and I was able to show her how to correct that. We added simple exercises to do at home that strengthen the muscles, ligaments, and tendons in her lower extremities (ankle, foot) to improve foot placement. Another problem for Jill was keeping alignment when she*

*was driving. Because she is petite, she had to overcom-*
*pensate for issues, like pedal length and chair height.*
*We were able to figure out what she needed to prevent*
*overcompensation and keep her posture and alignment*
*maintained. We also noticed while sitting Jill had become*
*victim to pelvic tilt at work. I showed her how to maintain*
*her belly-button-to-breastbone distance on her body*
*which has helped her low back and pelvic issues. I have*
*given her basic exercises to do at home daily that will*
*keep her strong and keep her in appropriate alignment.*
*In addition, we conducted a gait analysis to see if there*
*were any other fundamental issues. We found that Jill has*
*hypermobile joints, which leaves her prone to injury. KT*
*tape was another tool placed on certain parts of her body*
*to remind her of proper alignment.*

The tool used in this method is to "think in threes." Saying it will trigger a reminder to consider the right three steps
to take or systems to consider when trying to solve or remedy
an issue.

In solving performance, pain, or injury issues involved in
the musculoskeletal or the structure system, break it down into
three parts of the structure—legs, core, and arms. All three
parts are interconnected and interdependent, as are the three
systems of the body. Two legs, each separately connected into
the bottom of the core just to the outside of the "sitting" bones;
the core, including the three bones of the pelvis, the bones of
the lumbar and thoracic spine stacked on top, the discs

between, and twelve ribs connected on each side of the thoracic
spine and in the front at the
breastbone; two arms connected
on the shoulder blade to the outside of the armpit under the shoulder tip; and the shoulder tip
attached to the collarbone as the
only bony attachment of the
hand/arm to the remainder of the
body at the top of the breastbone.
Each bone is aligned with another
bone. Their surfaces are parallel to
each other. The place where bones
are connected are called joints.
The function of the joints is to
allow motion, but the shape of the
bone ends and the size and shape
of the muscles around the joints

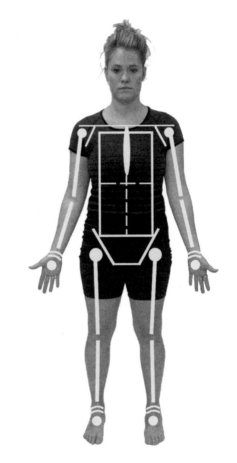

determine the direction and load the joint can handle. This
shape will determine what direction or directions the next joint
above or below it can move. This is a little like pushing a line
of dominoes. The angle of the first one pushed will determine
where the next one goes. This is how the sequence of movement is determined in your body. There is always the phenomenon of chain reaction in play when your body is being
supported and moved. Maintaining appropriate alignment in
any given situation is dependent upon the speed, force, and

endurance required to complete the task. Always a continuous factor is the force of gravity bearing down on our structure in relationship to the surface below us in tasks requiring both stillness and movement. Recognizing that your body must adjust, then learning how you can make changes to reset it in order to rest and recover or to make it more efficient to improve performance, is what the "think in threes" tool will provide for you. When you are successfully aligned, your muscles can create optimal loading through the bones and joints in order to move and support the body. This alignment at the joints is essential for providing effective circulation that brings nutrients and takes toxins away from the joints, muscles, and other tissues, and allows for best performance and recovery.

Although there are similarities to a machine, your body is, of course, organic, and changes with every step you take. As a sailor, I know that you cannot change the wind, but you can adjust your sails. While understanding your structure, you can adjust and change your body parts while also recognizing the things you cannot change. Understand that when designing vehicles and buildings, the measurements used are based on the average person's structural build and makeup; people who don't fit within the average building or vehicle may experience strains and stresses to their structure, unless they make intentional modifications to adapt to the reality. Rethink your expectations that the furniture, computers, and equipment change for you! Recognize that you can change and adjust equipment and furniture to work better for you. Understanding how each of the three body systems and parts adjust and adapt for each other's losses/weaknesses will allow you to develop a systematic way to assess your own health and maintain your musculoskeletal structural support to reset your body.

## Nutrition/Fluid/Gas System

The nutrition/fluid/gas system processes all inhaled and ingested substances and provides the other two systems the hydration and nutrition they need, while also removing waste. The circulation system is the nutrient transporter after the organs have liquefied and processed what you have eaten; then the other organs including the lungs process and remove waste and handle the chemical balancing act all dictated by the brain. If there is any lack of circulation of fluids/nutrients to a part of your structure, the brain will demand an adjustment to remedy this situation by shifting muscle use. If successful, the circulation will be restored, but the adjustments made will eventually catch up. The result can be muscle pain, feeling "tight," or spasms, due to toxin congestion that has not been washed out. Most muscular and skeletal pain and performance issues originate from congestion of toxic waste and decreased nutrient supply because of compression of joint surfaces that are covered with bone-end protective-cartilage covers embedded with sensors. In addition, the overused muscles create an overloading volume of toxins within the fascia surrounding the muscles, causing a pain alarm, forcing adjustment of muscle to keep the structure moving and upright. The pain or tightness warning is sounded throughout the body when there is imminent failure, such as tearing or breakdown of the compressed tissues, including cartilages or disc materials. For example, we know that the nerve (median) affected in carpal tunnel syndrome takes up to twenty-four hours for the swelling to resolve and to restore normal functioning after only twenty minutes of pressure on the wrist area. During the compression time and then for the twenty-four hours after you will notice stiffness, pain, and possibly a feeling of weakness. Your brain is giving you the signal that there is damage. The remedy is to recognize this as something you can prevent and resolve with intentional corrective reset body position change. The solution is simple and no new desk is generally necessary.

**Patient Story:** *Jane A.—Jane hobbled in, and walked out! She was taught the importance of intentionally learning how to reset her body to minimize stress and maximize performance. She had one treatment during which I explained the importance of circulation and that by crossing her legs she was cutting off her blood supply, which was needed for optimal mechanical advantage for the muscles.*

# Nervous System: Brain, "Wizard of Bod," and the Conscious Mind, Spinal Cord, and Nerves

The third and most important body system, the nervous system, includes the subconscious brain (or what I like to call the "Wizard of Bod"), the conscious mind, the decision maker, the spinal cord, and the nerves, or "wires," which conduct the informational data to and from the sensors throughout the body. The brain interprets data from sensors all over the body (the five senses) and then gives instruction and adaptations to the structure and fluid/nutrition/gas systems to allow the body to remain in homeostasis.

First you must understand the way you learn to move. When you are learning a new skill, such as a new dance, this is learned by watching and then mimicking the dance steps. Think about the first time you had to join a line dance. Hopefully, you did not shut your eyes! You used your visual senses to memorize the sequence to replicate the dance. The muscles do not remember the moves. The senses of touch, including sensors in the joints, record pressures needed in the joints in the exact time, speed, and force to replicate the goal activity, i.e., to be able to perform the new dance steps. The ligaments and the tendons have length sensors to give the brain tension information so that it knows how much force is needed to be recruited or to be released to allow and control the muscle use necessary to perform a task. It is not a function of strength or flexibility at this point. To demonstrate the fact that muscle memory is actually sensory memory or a sequence of muscle and joint use, which equals movement, complete the "Is It Muscle Memory?" worksheet on page 122. After you've finished completing the worksheet, consider what this exercise demonstrates. While writing with your opposite hand you may have noticed you write slower, couldn't push the pen with the same amount of force, or write with adequate precision. To get better at writing with your opposite hand you wouldn't complete strength exercises. Strength does not predict performance. In order to achieve the same results when writing with your opposite hand, you would need to practice the proper sequence of motion. Applying this to your body, strength is usually not the primary issue; instead you need to be able to replicate the movement pattern sequence correctly to perform your specific activity with the outcome you expected. As you found in the writing exercise, you certainly would not get better writing your name by lifting weights, would you?

Without the brain, the structure (the body and organs/vessels) and nutrient systems would not be able to function. The brain is the control center, but also dependent on the other two systems and vice versa. Without appropriate nutrients, which include all types of fluids and gases moving through your body or structure, over time, the brain will not function. The muscles are actually the primary stimulant to the body by helping keep the nutrients and waste moving efficiently and effectively throughout the body by staying active throughout the day. Failure in one system essentially results in failure to all. When you improve structure and health, you can expect improvement in all three systems because it directly correlates with the other two systems.

The brain learns movement over your lifetime. It memorizes routine activity sequences of movement such as walking,
sitting down, and standing up, through the sensory systems of
the muscle actions. Each of these patterns or sequences, when
repeated over time, are permanent. Until you have a need to
modify or adapt your movement sequence, such as when you
are learning a new sport, have an injury, or unintentionally stay
in an awkward position too long, your brain automatically sub-
consciously can repeat the previously learned movements or
positions. The structures and hydration and nutrition systems
depend upon instruction from the nervous system. When there
is a need to adjust the pattern or sequence of how or when to
move the body, you must first rethink what is happening to

Try this to demonstrate "choose to use" if your body is not aligned or
supported. Hold your head in a forward position, ears forward over
shoulder sockets. Note that your muscles in the back of your neck will
quickly fatigue. To understand how this problem is compounded with
failure to support your arm while you use your arm, hold a glass of water
(equal amount in each glass) in each hand with your elbows bent at a 90
degrees and thumbs pointing up. Keep one arm firmly against your side
and move the other arm and hand forward about 8 to 10 inches. Now
keep them still for one minute. Did one side tire earlier? The side unsupported and not lined up with the remainder of the body had to use more
muscle power because there was less support. The brain will have to send
more muscle power to the unsupported arm and neck muscles, therefore
fatiguing and causing pain faster.

make the change necessary, then recognize what you need to do to change. With practice and precision over time, you can reset the way you are aligned for successful goal attainment. It will not happen without these three steps.

**Patient Story:** *Mr. Thomas—Mr. Thomas, a former college athlete, is now a businessman approaching retirement as the owner of a heavy equipment company. He has limited his activities to walking in the dirt, climbing in and out of the heavy machinery, and watching his grandchildren play sports (one in college). He begrudgingly consulted with me, coming in with his daughter, who insisted he see me. He could barely walk without the assistance of a cane and support of his daughter due to severe pain in one of his hips. He had seen three doctors who had scanned and X-rayed him, and pronounced that there was nothing to do but wait until a total joint replacement was necessary. He was given a prescription for physical therapy and faithfully went to every visit. He was instructed in the "classic" leg raises and squats, and given heat and electric stimulation. As an athlete, he recognized the exercises he was asked to do, but they didn't seem appropriate or useful. As a businessman, he recognized that there was no common sense or sequence of planning with this approach to solving his problem. He did not understand any of his goals. But he was being asked to suspend his disbelief and just do what they said. No results. He did not improve with treatment and lost three* *months he could never get back. He had already been going to a gym and was regularly performing cardio and other exercises recovering from another issue, which none of the professionals he was working with seemed to recognize. On his return visit to his doctor, who had ordered the PT, he was offered drugs for the continuing pain and the new depression he was now experiencing. In addition, he was told, "Maybe you should try yoga. I really like it!" This roughly two-hundred-seventy-five-pound gentleman, with a self-proclaimed pot belly, looked at the doctor and said, "Really, Doc? Try to visualize me in a yoga class!" He walked away, not feeling heard or understood. He felt like his problems and goals had not been considered, let alone realistically addressed. His life was ticking by again with no plan that suited his needs. He recognized he was overweight (not a new issue), but his weight was getting rapidly worse from inactivity. He also recognized he had had plenty of injuries, including some big orthopedic surgeries. He was able to recover enough to keep doing the things he wanted to do. Pain was not new, but pain to this extreme level had stopped him in his tracks. On his first day in my office, with lots of encouragement and interviewing, he completed a history of all of his injuries and their outcomes, a job description, an everyday activity description including areas of difficulty (athletic play and self-care, such as putting on socks or climbing stairs) and a prioritized activity goal sheet. He was asked to demonstrate his general required everyday movements and we recorded him doing some of these activities, noting pain and positions he started in and the sequence of how he then used his body to both support and move him through the activities. One of the most seemingly simple activities he had trouble with was transitioning from sitting in a chair to standing. Looking at his recording performing the activity, drawing on his athletic abilities and knowledge of the "athletic position," helped him recognize his foot would drift to the outside just before he stood up. He could see his foot was not supporting his body. With a quick visual and tactile reset, he learned that if he first stopped and thought how he was setting up his leg positions both during sitting and standing and then recognized that his repeated loading in this way was damaging his joints (pain) and the muscles were not in a mechanically sound position because of this, then he was able to reset his body. In other words, by looking at the position of the joints of his legs to see the best alignment, then modifying to the best position, his ability to go from sitting to stand, and vice versa, was dramatically improved. He had not been able to do this pain-free for six months, and with his three-second reset he performed the movement pain-free! The same result occurred while addressing his wobbly, stiff, and painful walking. Rethinking the current movement sequence was causing undue compression on the tender part of his hip, resulting in a side-to-side "waddling" walk. He recognized this not only made him slower, but instead of going forward he was walking further and spending more time on the sore part of his hip: all ineffi-cient movement patterns and not the way bodies are designed to move. He recognized that this adaptation over a long period of time had finally caught up with him and caused pain. The solution was not more strength exer-cises, but rather rethinking what had happened to his movement sequence (use of muscles with the skeleton), and recognizing the sequence so he could reset his walk-ing. Mr. Thomas doesn't like to admit that he walked into my office with a cane and additional support, but that's okay. Now he is in a positive state of mind and has returned to his ability to enjoy his work and family. As a younger athlete, he had known the natural movement of his body and understood how far he could push through injuries and anything life threw at him. As time marched on, the solutions he was offered only fixed the conse-quences of his former improper movement patterns. Unfor-tunately, medical professionals only offered him surgery or drugs, nothing to alter his body to previous abilities through understanding the language of his own body and resetting through natural movements. Tapping into his history and abilities instead of ignoring them allowed for the restoration of his functioning abilities.*

Your subconscious brain, or your "Wizard of Bod," works continuously to make the necessary adjustments to help you survive, regardless of the activities you perform. And it gives you the language needed to understand and assess the changes of your body, and to adapt and adjust resources as needed. If there is a lack in one system, the brain directs resources and abilities from the other systems to help.

The brain has the ability to *rethink, recognize,* and then *reset,* while measuring the responses of your body. Pain is the language your Wizard of Bod uses to warn your body of impending harm, an alarm for your conscious, decision-making, and learning brain (neurologic, electrical control system) to pay attention and to encourage a change. It is a *positive* alarm, sounded only when there is imminent danger of injury or failure in one or more of your body systems. When the issue is not resolved, sensitivity to pain stimuli increases, and performance decreases. With stress, fear, or lack of understanding about potential procedures and outcomes, often altered with medication, the pain signals will get more frequent and intense. Opportunity to prevent injury, resolve perform-

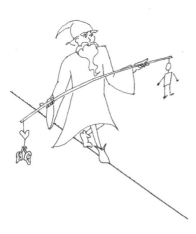

ance, and treat pain (stop meds!) is already within your body. Learn to listen to and understand the signals and alarms your brain is giving you. Learn to stop and recognize and differentiate the type of "pain" you are experiencing. Is it attached to a fear emotion? Is there an activity you have just performed, or a weather change that contributed to the feeling you now have? With patience and practice you can learn when the primary cause of musculoskeletal performance injury issue is secondary to a miscalculation in alignment.

The brain works all of the time during activities we do in our lives by
adjusting and adapting the three systems of our bodies to keep us moving. The conscious, decision-making
part of our brain is where we can
learn and understand how to change
preventable injuries and pain to
maintain optimal performance and
health for life even before the pain
alarm or performance potential is
altered. After you learn to reset your
body initially, you will be able to use
the three-step method for a lifetime.

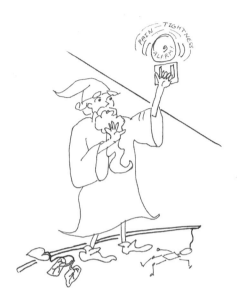

In order to move, you incorporate all five senses, as well
as common sense. Movement occurs by a most optimal muscle
sequence used for every task each time it is performed. Movement is performed by muscle actions on the bone attachments.
The sequence, position, timing, and load is determined after
the brain evaluates information from the senses, primarily
sight and touch. The brain acquires about eighty percent of its
information from the eyes to either learn or relearn a movement. Pressure sensors in the ends of the bones at the joints
tell the brain how much load is on the joint, the sensors in the
ligaments and tendons report the tension on these structures
so the brain knows how much force is needed, and the skin,
the largest organ of the body, provides a vast amount of information to the brain regarding the surface type—hard or soft,

hot or cold—and angle to help the brain determine the combination of muscles to recruit in order to attain then maintain optimal alignment, weight, load, speed, and position to successfully complete the task requirements. The brain acquires eighty percent of its information from the eyes to determine what muscles are needed to recruit and execute an activity. The brain—not the muscles—eventually memorizes the muscle sequence, including the weight, speed, and range of motion necessary to perform the activity. The chain reaction or sequence of transferring and controlling the body weight through support and movements is somewhat like a chess game, and is often referred to as the kinetic chain. If an adjustment is necessary because of a disabled part from injury or disease, the subconscious brain will seek an immediate and most convenient revised sequence of muscle use to accomplish the goal. These adjustments are generally not sustainable over a long time because the substitution parts were not designed for these jobs. There are not an infinite number of adjustment combinations of muscles available. There are not replacement parts when repair can no longer keep up with the demands of the body. When all possible adjustments have been used in a body, then pain and breakdown will ensue. (We will go into more detail about the systems breaking down later in this book.) The majority of issues in musculoskeletal injury and performance are secondary to unsustainable adjustments over time causing breakdowns of the tissues. But these breakdowns are usually reversible and entirely treatable!

**Guidelines to Maintain Best Circulatory and Electrical (Nervous System) Function:**

- Keep ankle at or less than a 90-degree position.
- Keep knees bent no more than 90 degrees while seated.
- Keep thighs apart in a "V" position.
- Upper arms should be supported and 20 degrees away from side seam.
- Keep shoulders from shrugging and ears over shoulder tips.

## Rethink, Recognize, Reset

The three-step method is designed to use simple assessments, planning, and implementation steps, providing reproducible tools, skills, and tips to help you reach your performance potential. The method is the application for solving the most common and predictable body issues. These three steps— rethink, recognize, and reset—will help you predict, attain, and maintain optimal health and performance, including pain

Most of my patients worry about going on a summer vacation to Europe or New York because of the increased amount of walking. Rarely is the extra walking really a problem. In fact, they always feel better. More movement increases circulation to maintain hydration to the brain, joints, and muscles.

control, preventing injuries, and reaching goals in athletic/ fitness, work, and/or daily performance. This book is intended to get you started at the very basic level. Use it first to try to solve your most fundamental issues. Prioritize solving the most important issue. What is affecting your quality of life the most? Through well-verified science, there is evidence that most all muscle and joint issues can be improved upon and/or resolved if we approach them with a correct method. Maybe consider these issues for example: Do you wake up with a stiff neck? Have you been going to the same health provider or classes but not getting better? Did you start having low back soreness after sitting on an airplane for two hours? Does your shoulder get sore after or during a swim? Have you turned down an opportunity to join a friend in an activity because you thought you could not keep up or were worried you would have pain? This method provides a three-step blueprint to help you interpret the language of your body and take the right three steps to reach your optimal potential.

# Step One: Rethink

Step one is to rethink the issue(s) involved. Rethinking is a reminder to have reflection time and to actually stop and carefully listen to what your body is telling you. Start with defining and describing what your issue is, even if it is a re-injury. Make sure you know exactly what body parts are at play and recognize how it affects your other systems as well (i.e., lack of sleep, overeating, fear, relationship issues, increased anxiety, etc.). Be mindful what happens to your pain or symptoms when you change to different positions throughout the day. Once you know what the issues are, write clear and concise goals that pertain to your specialized and specific activities (work, everyday tasks, and play/athletic performance). Finally, you will need to identify your solution team members you have been using and what you have been using as solutions and the outcomes to date. You will learn to read and interpret the language of your body, understanding both what is normal, natural movement as opposed to altered positions and movement sequences you have defaulted into.

**Patient Story:** *Margaret Moore—After seven years of knee pain with few good answers and little relief from orthopedic physicians, other physical therapists, and* *"wellness" doctors, Margaret came to me. Having been a Division I athlete and a lifetime runner she was beyond frustrated to be dealing with severe knee pain in her early forties. My approach was simple and yet unlike anything any other professional had told her. I suggested to her that the most basic movements, such as the way our feet strike the ground and propel us forward, are critical to the over-all health of our bodies. It's easy to think that sort of thing is second nature, but often we must reteach our bodies how to sit, stand, and walk properly to avoid chronic pain. Margaret is now virtually pain free without medications, injections, braces, or any other "crutches." Any occasional pain is brought on because she needs to reset her alignment. She has recently brought her own middle- and high-school age children to me to have them evaluated and educated.*

## Identify and Verify Your Issues

The first step of rethinking is to define and confirm the individual issues needing to be addressed by listing and prioritizing them. Try to be realistic about the importance of how each issue affects your quality of life and your potential for best health for a lifetime. A new consult or assessment might be necessary during this step. As I stated earlier, the number one criteria to predict success when attaining a goal is to most accurately and expediently acquire the root cause of your pain or issue. Without either the appropriate diagnosis and/or clarifying of the scope of the issue and modifying expectations as needed, a waste of time, money, and even worsening or no results can be the outcome. It is so hard to be patient moving through completion of this step, but it is essential if you truly want to reach and maintain your best body health and use for a lifetime. Start with stating your issue: for example, waking up with stiffness on the right side of your neck, causing restriction in rotation every morning for the first two hours of the day. As you become more skilled using the three-step method as a tool, you will be able to tackle more complex issues.

Write down three issues that you would like to address with the three-step method starting with your top priority.

## Goal Setting

Be realistic setting goal expectations. Again, we are beginning in the basic mode. Requirements include attaching measurement and time to your goals. In the next step of the method, there will be an assessment of where exactly to start and a fine tuning of your plan. However, you must have a realistic goal in order to know if the plan you have implemented, the money you have spent, or the class you have taken has been effective. These are *your* goals, not your coaches' or health provider's. To begin, a goal could be: drive to and from work every day without pain by the end of four weeks. That goal fulfills the goal setting requirements of measurement and time for assessment. Too often, patients put "pain free" on their goal sheet, but fail to put any terms of measurement. Unfortunately, life is never entirely pain free, and as stated earlier, occasionally we all get hurt, but most injuries heal if we let them. Another common goal patients write down is to "run better." Again, this has no measurable component or time for attaining the goal. Try changing your goal to: Run two miles at an average of eight minutes per mile, four days per week, within seven weeks. That fulfills all the criteria. Without the measurability and time for completion, there is no end to the treatment or training and no accountability for the trainer or exercise instructors or medical or health provider. Please read that as lost time and lost potential for you. Get rid of the most defeating issue in successful goal attainment: letting *hope* trump *reality*. Realism in goal-setting must be relative to many factors, including your current conditioning, if an athletic or performance goal, and when you are planning to participate in a competition. It might also be in relation to a medical diagnosis. I have treated hundreds of patients living with Amyotrophic Lateral Sclerosis (ALS) through Johns Hopkins Hospital for nearly ten years. I learned so much from each and every one of my patients, and I am eternally grateful to all of them. Goal-setting and attention to relevance was one of those lessons I learned. The average time a person with ALS would live after receiving a definitive diagnosis is eighteen months. So, when I, as a member of the solutions team, would meet them shortly thereafter; they would quickly let me know their goals were number one, to beat the disease, and number two to strengthen muscles to stop the advancement of the disease. This is an extreme example where hope had beaten reality, meaning the reality was and is that there is no cure. I was responsible for helping them understand and reset their goals to maintain the highest level of optimal health for their lifetime.

Other examples pop up in sports participation planning, which include an understanding that if you are from a family with an average height of five-feet-five inches, a goal to be an NBA basketball player will probably end in disappointment. A more realistic goal would include a better match for the size and structure you have been given and learning how to enhance and take care of your body over your lifetime rather than expecting breakdown. The issue and solutions should answer these questions:

1. What is wrong with you? Not simply a list of results of what you have been doing.
2. What will the provider do for you specifically? Expect and request valid researched rationales.
3. What can you do for yourself? This includes your limitations and precautions.
4. What is the expected outcome? What is the expected time line, and how will this be measured and or modified? This should include your long-term goals and short-term goals.

Understand and seek common sense approaches from your solution team members. Look at the big picture attached to your goals and ask the professionals and providers to focus on teaching you what the relevance of a test result is on either your potential to improve, or need to modify or change your plan of action in solving your issues. This will allow you to move forward in proper sequences. I urge patients to keep a realistic reference to their goal expectations related to their own and family injury and health history. Keep in mind that health is defined by the World Health Organization as "a resource for everyday life, not an objective of living; it is a positive concept emphasizing social and personal resources as well as personal capabilities" (Duthey, 2013). I recommend you do not define your expectations solely by the outcomes of your relatives' health care but to learn the past successes or failures in yourself and family members that includes sensitivity to medications or foods, propensity to immune reactions, response to pain stimuli, and healing speed. Remember you can learn from the past, but now understand how to optimize your own health for the future using the three-step method resetting your body resources.

Goal setting is a vital part of recognizing your issue. To improve upon, attain, or maintain expected outcomes for any one of the goals or reasons that compelled you to pick up and use this book—change pain, injury, and/or work or athletic performance—it is essential to follow a process. This sets up the appropriate basis for solution planning, including the what, how, and when to implement appropriate tools and skills. Think about it: if you want to relieve pain, you need to attach relevant, realistic, and measurable activities as a basis to monitor progress toward success. There are tons of apps on your phones, iPads, etc., to record and measure and track progress toward your goals. Those resources are not the issue. The issue is: how do you know how to set up, reset, or modify the goal? "Get rid of pain," "do better in lacrosse," or "stop spraining my ankle," are not measurable goals.

Are your goals realistic? Compare the details of the cause of the issues being addressed with the goal activities being reset in this program. Consider the implication of your history both with past attempts at solving a similar issue and the realities of your own potential to reach the goals you are setting. It is not a mystery where your structure comes from or what we can expect from it. Scientific evidence with DNA, your genes, and history dictate structure features and performance potentials. You have attained your structure from your parents and their parents. You have inherited their sizes, shapes, performance capabilities and breakdown potentials. Your expectations of your goal potential must be based on the reality of your inherited potential, then enhance and care for yourself for optimal outcomes. While goal setting, you recognize the realities of past use of your structure and develop realistic expectations moving forward. Only after this is it possible to plan how to reach those goals. Consider thinking in terms of how you would maintain a car. Would you purchase a car in the year that you were born, not do any maintenance, and expect it to work the same forty years later and cost nothing to restore and maintain? We seem to have that expectation of our bodies, especially our structure. We seem universally surprised when we have broken-down backs and knees when we are in our thirties and forties, seemingly unable to accept the connection with the additional twenty-five to forty pounds gained, previous injuries, more sedentary lifestyle, coupled with poor posture all compounded with time. Again, using the car example: with a history of multiple accidents, use of wrong fuels, not repairing alignment problems, the car would, understandably, have poor performance, undependable usage, and the cost to restore it would take time and significant effort. Some issues may not be completely reparable. A successful coach once said that he had more success with his team when he spent time optimizing best form, mobility, and agility with average athletes and team performance versus only focusing on the few exceptional, so-called "natural" athletes. In addition, recognize that although humans have the same general number of body parts, these entities frequently vary in shapes and sizes, but can usually be managed with appropriate body care and attention. Husain Bolt, for example, has a half-inch leg length difference and scoliosis, but happens to be the fastest man in the world, with eight Olympic gold medals and twenty-eight career medals to prove it. He does not use a heel lift for his leg discrepancy. He focused on what he could do rather than on the issues with his body structure. Ability is greater than disability. Having flat feet does not necessarily mean that orthotics will be necessary to adapt for the collapsed arch within the foot. Curves of the spine vary quite a bit between people and are subject to varying strains from muscular control imbalances. A medical professional should identify the unique articulations of a person's body structure and tailor recovery toward the specific demands and daily activities the individual engages in. Be wary of a one-size-fits-all approach.

After considering this information, it's time to define your goals. The process must be repeated every time a new issue emerges. How will you know if you are progressing? How will you know if the assessment modifications skills, tools, and professionals you are using to attain and or maintain your goals are appropriate or adequate?

Think in threes. The three essential components of goal setting are:

1. Accurate assessment and/or diagnosis of the issue. Instead of saying "low back pain," rethink and use "muscle spasm in the right side of back after ten minutes of being seated at my computer."
2. Develop goals that are measurable. For example, instead of "stop pain while sitting at my computer," try: No pain (0) on 0–5 scale when sitting at my computer at home for more than thirty minutes.
3. Prioritize the goals in order of importance to you. I recommend that you try to have one goal in each of the three categories as appropriate: play/athletics, work performance, everyday activities for connecting the other activities (driving, laundry, shopping, etc.).

Complete the Activity Goal Sheet on page 126. I highly recommend, even if you are only working in a basic mode at this point, that you complete the Patient Specific Activity

(PSAS) score for at least one goal. This is the one valid measurement score to assess progress and assessment of abilities discussed later.

## Choosing Your Solution Team Members

If you need additional help to attain your goal, either to identify your issues and/or implement your plan of action to reset your body, you will need to complete this step to assess the effectiveness of what you have tried in the past and determine if the team members are the right choices for you. There are emerging concepts about how to develop the most effective team. Most currently there is evidence that to solve pain issues, the team members must be kept to a minimum. Three is optimum. This team number will change as your needs and goals are attained and changed. Again, keep in mind that this book is addressing basic changes to structure, but these changes can be very powerful. I have seen someone's potential ruined by well-meaning excessiveness with too many doctors, therapists, and exercise routines. The time, money, and overall stress in coordinating all of these therapies can sabotage the healing effects that might have occurred.

In addition, be wary of excessive talk, especially in medical terms, by the members within your solutions team. Your team should reflect people and tools with the relevant and validated experience in your area of goal needs.

It is also vitally important to understand the meaning of credentials, licensure, and certifications. Credentials consist of the list of certifications and licensures the person has earned. To become more efficient and effective in your efforts for success, look up the requirements for the certifications and licensures your team members list. Understand the requirements for certifications are not mandated, validated, or controlled by anyone beyond the group who invented the certification class. Therefore, there is no legal protection for the consumer, or consistent knowledge requirements from one certification to the next even within the same category (for example, personal training or pilates). Understand the level of education required that has been validated; i.e., a college degree from an accredited university versus classes held in a setting and developed outside this system. Licensure mandates legally binding standards of minimal education, training, and retraining, and provides the consumer protection from misuse of the services, standards, and ethics of the provider. Simply stated, although every profession (a job which requires advancing skill sets and education versus a job that includes voluntary education and no mandated consumer protection) has members who are better at their skills than others. Be wary of instant cures, fancy language, and "too good to be true" solutions by a team member, especially if their only credentials are those attained without sanctioned, validated education and training. Redundant care to help manage your health by different professionals often leads to excessive spending both of time and money. In addition, think in threes to remember that working with no more than three people at one time during activity goal attainment generally is enough. Consider phasing goals and possibly phase team members in and out of your primary solution team to most accurately assess effectiveness of each member at the time. Money is best spent, and results are reached faster, with a realistic set of goals, and fewer, but most effective, team members possible, using the most proven tools and skills relevant to your issues. Before moving forward, understand the team, tools, and skills you are using currently so that you can streamline, validate, and not replicate. Complete the Solutions Team 1 & 2 Worksheets in the Toolbox on pages 128–131.

On completion of the Solution Team 1 & 2 Worksheets, review the redundancy and clarify who, how, what, and when each team member's tools and skills you will need to use. This stage begins to determine how to implement your plan of action to reach your goals. Again, if you are starting in the basic mode, I would recommend you complete this form, and consider using this as a tool for organizing your health-care team for general health needs. Share the solution team you have chosen with your primary care physician. If you do not already have one for an annual physical, consider finding one and use this form to sort out credentials when you are vetting friends and family recommendations, so you can avoid being trapped into the hope versus reality category.

# Step Two: Recognize

## Learning Alignment

Recognizing your proper alignment is the second step of aligning for success in this three-step method. This second step uses the application of the "think in threes" tool to focus on joint position at the basic level to make sure that all structure segments can be, and are, appropriately aligned. If a new issue arises, measure progress to adjust for modification needs along the way. To begin any and all skills tests you always need to assess the body from the ground up, starting with the feet. Remember: practice and patience are mandatory. Small changes will often make a big difference. Be very disciplined to start from the feet upward, even if you are trying to solve a neck issue. After all, your neck is at the top of all of the bones teetering above a large stack of other bones balanced by muscles constantly being adjusted by your brain, while you are often mindlessly unsupported, losing sleep, poorly hydrated, overexercising . . . you get the picture! It's now time to recognize your own alignment so that you can assess and reset it.

Think in threes: legs, core, upper body. Refer to your Geography of Your Structure Worksheet for geographical landmarks. Having a mirror is recommended because your brain needs eyes to assess the situation. Have someone take a picture or record this session for you to review and compare later. Use the Alignment Checklist found in the Toolbox (page 123) to both record what you find to complete the three-step method, and also use again if you have an issue in the future.

The most important part is the base of support: your feet!

Try these practices below:

# Legs

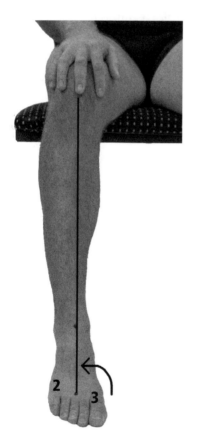

## Foot and ankle alignment, sitting (bare feet)

Using three fingers on the kneecap, confirm that middle finger is aiming straight down to the mid-ankle and base of third toe. If not, move your forefoot, arrow at mid-foot, and/or knee position to align properly. Toes are flat and three points of foot have even pressure.

Place three fingers on your knee cap. Your middle finger should shoot down and connect to your mid-ankle joint and base of the third toe. Make sure you pull your arch up. No matter how far apart the thighs are or direction they are facing, this is always the same check. Each leg is separately confirmed. Each foot should have equal weight distributed between the underside of outside of the heel (#1), under the base of the little toe (#2) and big toe (#3). Tripod foot support. Toes flat, not bent.

## Foot and ankle alignment, standing (bare feet)

Using three fingers on the kneecap, confirm that middle finger is aiming straight down to the mid-ankle and base of third toe. If not, move your forefoot, arrow at mid-foot, and/or knee position to align properly. Toes are flat and three points of foot have even pressure.

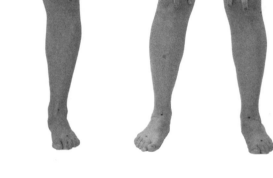

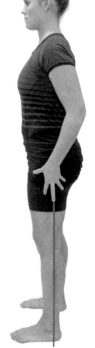

Correct                                        Incorrect

## Feet, hips alignment, from side

Finding alignment: With three fingers on side hip bone, confirm that middle finger is aiming straight toward the middle of the knee joint and the outside ankle bone. The line will be perpendicular to the floor.

## Hips, bending

Finding alignment: Widen the width of your legs and allow for a wider base when bending making sure thighs "V" from the center.

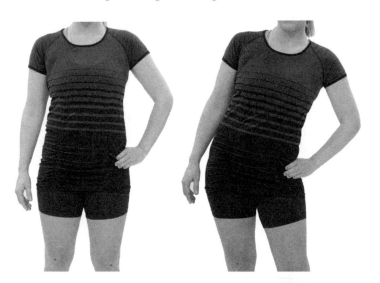

(above left) Finding top of leg (greater trochanter): Starting from top of pelvis, slide down until you feel the top of your leg bone. Place the web of your hand on top, your index finger at your hip crease and thumb resting toward the back of your body.

(above right) Confirming greater trochanter by side bending: With hand position described, bend over to the same side to confirm the web of your hand is in the crease made at the top of your leg bone. This will confirm your index finger will be resting over your ball-and-socket joint of your hip.

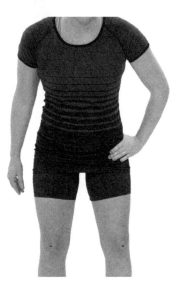

(right) Confirm appropriate thigh width for squatting and sitting. With your hand resting in the position found previously, adjust thigh width to maintain even pressure on all parts of the hand—web, thumb, and index finger—to avoid compression and injury in the hip joint. TIP: spread thighs wider as you bend your hips.

## Core: Pelvis, Sitting

Finding Alignment: Make sure your seat bones are even on right and left by checking with your three finger check described previously. Also, check to make sure they maintain even alignment when you change positions from sit to stand.

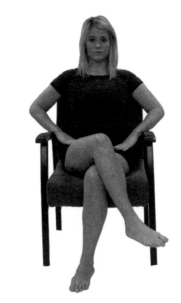

# Core

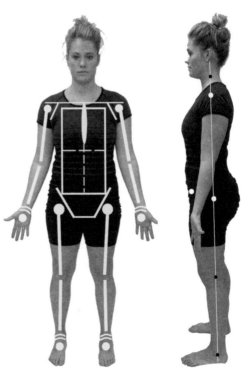

## Pelvis, standing

Finding Alignment: Make sure and check to see if your front pelvis bones are level.

## Ribs/spine, moving

Finding Alignment: Make sure all four quadrants are squared. Make sure you maintain the distance between the breastbone to belly button.

# Upper Body

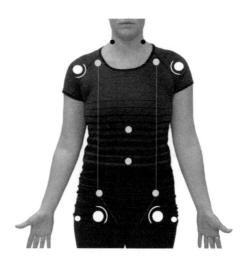

### Arms: Hands/Wrist

Finding Alignment: Make sure your middle finger (knuckle) is aligned with the mid-wrist and forearm.

### Elbow

Finding Alignment: Make sure the elbow is straight and not hyperextended. Make sure center elbow crease and center of wrist crease are aligned.

### Shoulders

Finding Alignment: Make sure that the biceps are forward and shoulder tip is below ear hole. Lift the top of the breastbone slightly if the shoulder tips are not aligned under the ears. Then gently pull the elbows toward your sides to allow the latissimus dorsi to activate and connect to the lower half support of the body. Also, make sure the shoulders are level, matching the hip level. Always lower the shoulder that looks higher. Latissimus dorsi are the muscles that perform this job, so pull slightly more with the elbow on the high shoulder side, toward your waist to help pull the shoulder level straight down. Do not fight gravity or change core forward or backward. This is a job for the shoulder blade.

## Head/neck, sit or stand

Finding Alignment: Place your thumb at your ear opening and then place your index finger at the nose tip and make sure your hand placement is level to the floor. Your elbows should be out.

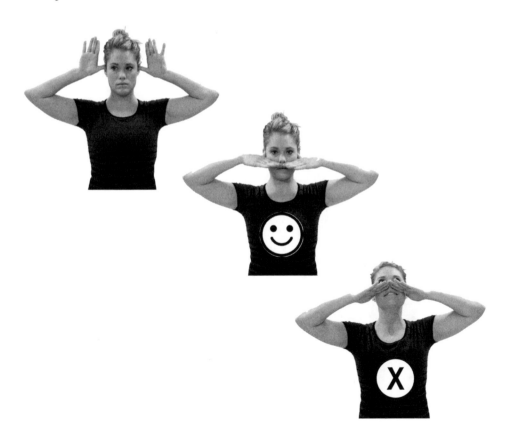

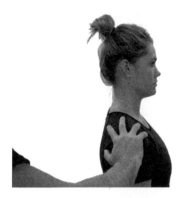
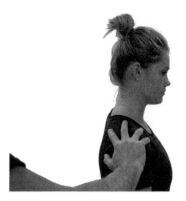

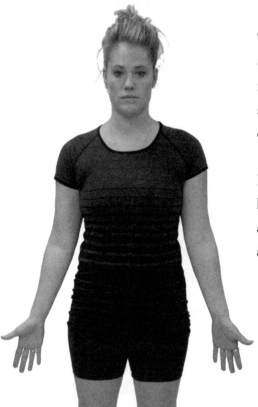

To confirm alignment of the shoulders, head, and neck, place your middle finger on your shoulder. It should then point directly to your ear opening.

Finding Alignment: Make sure your head and neck are even side to side and your ears are level both right and left.

# Establishing a Baseline

The *recognize* step of assessment is designed to help you prioritize the order to follow in resetting your body and reaching your goals. First, assess joint position, because without proper alignment the body may not be supported in your activities. If you cannot get into appropriate alignment you may need to see a physical therapist or other professional to assess why you cannot. I have included some commonly helpful activities and exercises that can help attain alignment in the Toolbox.

The second step of recognizing joint position is seeing if you can maintain the joint position in appropriate alignment. Obviously, without this ability, you will be at a higher risk for predictable syndromes and performance shortfalls, as we will point out later. Alignment at the joints and ability to maintain this position, both when still and throughout movement, eliminates compression on the ends of bones, straining of muscles, and balances muscle use. When the segments are properly aligned with or without weight, the joints of the body are mechanically advantaged to move proficiently and effectively. This creates immediate strength, called *structural strength*. Better performance in all activities is immediate when structure is optimally aligned. This also gives the tissues the opportunity to heal properly from regular use, previous injury, damage, or movement adaptation that may have occurred.

On completion of the Alignment Checklist (page 123) you will learn your own abilities, understand where your problem areas are in each of the three parts of your structure, and know where to reset to attain optimal body performance. Remember that your brain needs as much input as possible from your eyes and touch, so do have someone take a picture, record you, or just use a mirror to enhance your visualization and understanding of what needs to be reset in the plan. Try prioritizing what to work on by the most obvious part in each of the three segments of the structure, and reset each of those first. Rerecord how you are doing; periodically compare to your first recording and you will see progress. Reassess your patient specific ability score (PSAS) found on your Goal Sheet (page 126) and see if there has been a change.

# Make a Plan, Revise Goals and Solution Team Member Roles

After reviewing the results of the Alignment Checklist, update the Solutions Team Member list as needed as you assess the effectiveness and roles of your potential team members. For example, you might not understand or be able to hold a joint position, or possibly you have pain in another joint when you get to the position on your worksheet. You may need to consult with a physical therapist or your physician to assess how to proceed to reach your goals. Complete Team 1 & 2 Worksheets (pages 128–131) if there is a modified team member or change in their roles. This tool can also be used and modified in the staged phased in/out approach, but is a little more complicated. Use this form repeatedly to help when unexpected issues arise in the future.

# Develop a Plan

I am sure this seems overwhelming, and you might be thinking "let's just do it!" But as discussed earlier, the just "doing it" without taking the essential steps to develop a blueprint, or a road map for success, will end in lower results. Keep in mind when using this method, the more skill and understanding of how and when to use the tools will allow you to keep more of the activities you love and enjoy, such as gardening, running, or biking, and in most cases, will provide a way to return to activities you gave up in the past.

Think in threes: prioritize from your goal sheet and the results of your Alignment Checklist the alignment issue you need to work with first, especially related to the activity with which you have been having issues. This book is intended to teach the concepts of alignment and alignment resetting, primarily for basic activities (sit, stand, and reach). That said, you certainly could apply this concept or have your fitness and health professionals adapt this for you to continue building your skill for other movements. In the plan section of the Alignment Checklist, record how you will reset each of the joints you assessed as needing attention. It can be as simple as setting an alarm at your desk as a reminder to check posture every twenty minutes; K-taping right shoulder as a reminder to stop elevating it when you reach for your coffee cup; asking your spouse to say "sit up!" every time he/she sees you slouching. Place a reminder on your calendar to recheck your Alignment Checklist to see how you are doing in four weeks.

Reassess the PSAS and pain score on the Goal sheet and see how you are doing in four weeks. Make a commitment to at least check and commit to modify and seek answers if you are not any better or if you are progressing slower than you expected.

# Step Three: Reset Your Body

▲

## Implement the Plan: Putting It All Together

The third and final step of the three-step method is to *reset*. The reset step in the method is the implementation of body solutions. Patience, consistent systematic learning then applying of the "think in threes" tool in your goal activities, and applying the knowledge of how to listen to your body, will help you attain and maintain your goals and give you the freedom to participate in life. The key is to remember to focus on the joint alignment issues you saw during the assessment in the Alignment Checklist during your goal activities, but rapid success will occur if you remember to apply the skilled use of this tool in all activities of your life. Because you are functioning in a world with gravity and the most common issues occur when you are paying the least amount of attention to body alignment, there is a higher risk of injury.

## Resetting Joint Position

The "think in threes" tool is always applied from the feet upward to reset your body. The steps are as follows:

1. Take three seconds to check if each joint (exception below) is positioned in appropriate alignment. If you feel strain, then move your feet first to relieve strain. Continue changing each joint until you find relief. When you have learned your own appropriate alignment, and have become confident in applying it to resetting your body, you can use and reuse the Joint Positions (JP) Checklist in the Appendix to guide your reset as necessary.

2. Modify your environment and/or equipment involved in the task or position to maintain appropriate alignment. Remember you are the only thing that you can control and adjust. It is your responsibility.

3. Support your body structure in three points from the bottom half (below belly button and three points above) when possible to conserve muscle use and allow joints, muscles, and other structures recovery and repair throughout each day.

Reassessment of abilities is used to determine progress toward goals or effectiveness of interventions.

## General Reset Practice Session

This session is to help you understand positions and movements that are commonly involved with performance and injury issues:

# Applying Three-Step
# Method to Life

▲

## Confirming Appropriate Alignment – Advanced

**Foot-to-Hip Alignment**

Check and connect the dots of each leg segment separately regardless of which way the thigh is aiming (there are two hip socket holes). Knees should be straight in alignment while standing. From the side, the side hip bone, center of the knee, and side ankle bone should make a straight line. Move your foot first to reset knee position before moving knee.

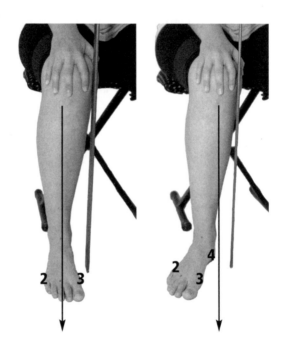

## Foot Alignment

Foot is comprised of three parts: rear, mid, and forefoot. The sequence of optimal use of the foot is dependent upon appropriate alignment. Because of this sequence, it is essential to reset the foot's ability for alignment from the rear to the forefoot. If the rear foot is not aligned, the next step in the sequence cannot be optimal and can affect the entire structure of the body. Thinking in threes as applied to foot alignment creates a reproducible method to check for alignment and then train the foot. The rear foot is the point of initial contact with both walking and running (more forward if running). As the body weight becomes supported, it is transferred to the mid foot, responsible for foot structure adjusting to uneven surfaces using side-to-side movements, shock absorption, and mobility. Finally, the sequence to transport the body's weight forward is the forefoot with toes critical for optimal propulsion.

## Hip Alignment

Find the top of leg by starting from top of pelvis, sliding down until you feel the top of your leg bone. Place the web of your hand on top, your index finger at your hip crease and thumb resting toward the back of your body. Confirm 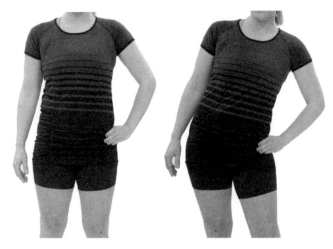 top of leg bone by side bending with hand position described, maintained, bend over to the same side to confirm the web of your hand is in the crease made at the top of your leg bone. This will confirm your index finger will be resting over your ball-and-socket joint of your hip.

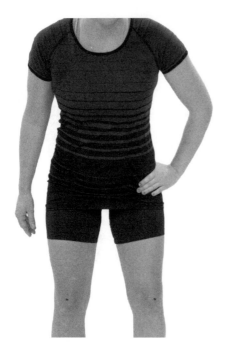

Confirm width for squatting, sitting. With your hand resting in the position found previously, adjust thigh width to maintain even pressure on all parts of the hand—web, thumb, and index finger to avoid compression and injury in the hip joint. TIP: spread thighs wider as you bend your hips. Keep hip angle in an open position as often as possible especially when driving and sitting at work to avoid compression of nerves, labrum, and other important circulation and support structures. The rule is that as the thigh gets closer to the chest, such as when you sit down or bring your knee toward your chest if lying down, you must have your thighs wider apart to avoid eventual degenerative joints and/or pain. Using "think in threes," practice finding the place on your hip crease where the hip joint is most relaxed and allowed to maintain appropriate circulation and support of all structures. An alternate method to find and practice confirming and resetting hip joint angles is using rulers. Find the hip joint with a ruler by sliding ruler up thigh until finding crease (often different angles side to side).

## Core

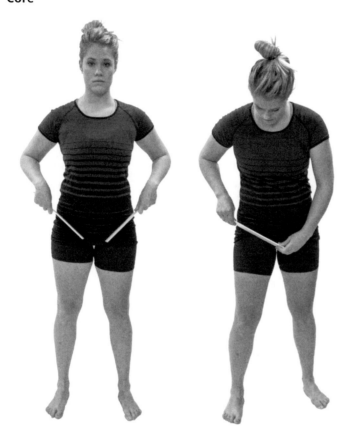

Confirming hip joint angle using rulers. Regardless of the direction of the thigh, the angle remains essentially unchanged. Find the hip joint with ruler by sliding ruler up thigh until finding crease (often different angles side to side).

The core consists of the ribs, breastbone, spine, and pelvis bones; it starts at the first rib and ends at the seat bones. The core contains four quadrants. The lats connect the top of the body to the bottom half of the body. Think of the core as a six-sided rectangle with the difference being that the arm and leg movements are not squared connections, but angled, dictated by the angle of the hip joints and the shoulder blade movement on the rib cage. Both are roughly thirty or so degrees and vary

from person to person. This angle allows the diagonal necessary for natural movement that resets fluids within the joints,
muscles, and other tissues essential for the body's optimal
performance and health. The connecting muscles crisscross on
the core on all six sides and are kept hydrated by our movement. Without appropriate maintenance of core alignment and
proper movement sequence of the arms and legs from one arm
to opposite leg in our day-to-day activities, we can expect less
performance and lower health than our potential. The latissimus dorsi muscles connect the top of the body to the bottom
half of the body. The core is a semi-stiff base of support to
allow movement of the arms above and legs below, and organ
function and protection within.

Throughout all your activities you will need to maintain
the appropriate distance between your belly button and breastbone at all times to ensure a safe spine and body function and
performance. This distance is found most accurately when you
lie on your back, knees bent comfortably with feet flat, then
lift arms over head as you inhale, exhale one or two times. Your
spine should now be relaxed to its natural appropriate position.
You can then use your hand as a measurement tool to check
for proper distance during all activities. Use this same hand
position to ensure that when you move your arms, you are also
maintaining the upper ribs still. The core is best maintained
when you move in proper sequence in all activities throughout
every day.

## Arms and Head/Neck

The arms hang from the muscles connected to the neck and head. The arm bones are attached to the remainder of the body only at the breastbone and collarbone junction. The latissimus dorsi is the muscle that not only primarily holds your spine upright, but also attaches to the front of your upper arm, then goes under your armpit, attaching to your shoulder blade, to your spine all the way to the base, and onto your pelvis bones. It is the muscle that keeps your arm from migrating up into your ears! The balance of muscular control is determined by appropriate alignment and support. The nerves and blood and lymph vessels all go under and through your collarbone and into your armpit and are vulnerable to being affected by adjustments necessary from inappropriate alignment and support. To confirm alignment of the shoulders, head, and neck, place your middle finger on your shoulder. It should point directly to your ear opening.

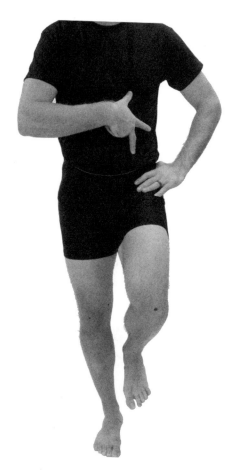

Confirming core and hip position with hip flexion.

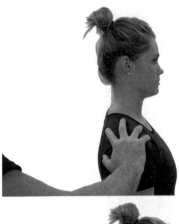

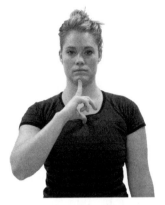

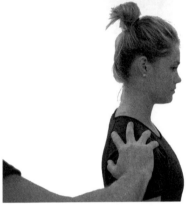

Confirming Head and Neck position: make an "L" with your hand and place your index finger on your chin and extend thumb to your chest; this is the distance that should be maintained between the head and the neck.

To confirm alignment of the arms and shoulders make sure the upper trapezius and ribs are quiet. The latissimus dorsi and abdominals are slightly contracted, and the shoulder blades should move on the ribs. The distance between the first rib and ear should never change. (See Alignment Checklist on p. 123.)

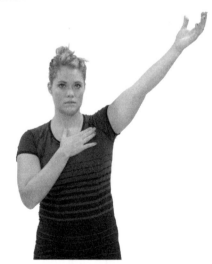

Confirming No Rib Movement: place hand on top of core then move arm over head or in any position of reach and confirm there is no rib movement throughout this arm motion.

# Applying Three-Step Method: Practice

## Common Activities

Let's Practice: Take a picture of yourself then use the Alignment Checklist (p. 123) to identify where you need to reset and modify. After completing the checklist, review each of the sections, then start resetting your body from the ground up, using the "think in threes" tool. Focus on the one joint that was the most difficult to correct first in each of the three sections instead of trying to correct absolutely everything at one time. Then as you learn to correct those joints, reassess and now correct the next problem. Practice the reset and rerecord or take more pictures to confirm how you have progressed. Always practice the part of the movement that you have been performing in an adapted position and as soon as you are able to control the joint in appropriate alignment, speed the movement to the speed you will be performing it in your everyday life.

## 1. Sitting

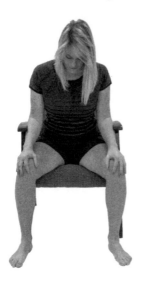
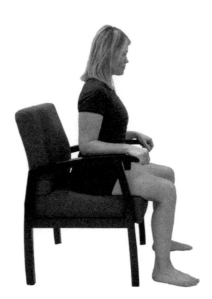

Think in threes and place hands on knee cap to check if feet, ankle and knee are in correct position, plus have feet the width of chair to ensure safe hip alignment. Choose to use the back support or arms of chair or even using thigh support with elbows (below) when you have it.

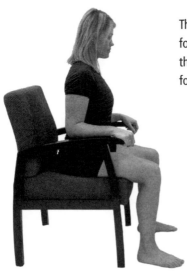

This is an alternate appropriate alignment for seated postures. Note the "think in threes" rules from feet up are all being followed.

## 2. Sit to Stand.

To build endurance, practice on a daily basis with the goal of
ten repetitions in ten seconds.

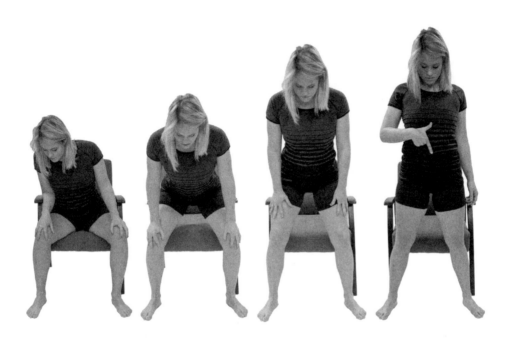

1. Confirm feet, ankle, and knee are in appropriate alignment.
2. Lean forward maintaining alignment.
3. Stand all the way the up, making sure the belly button to breastbone is maintained.

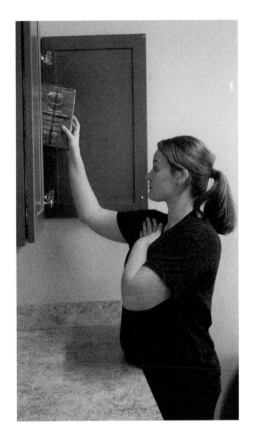

### 3. Reaching and lifting.

Confirm that your legs and core are maintained in appropriate alignment and that ear over shoulder tip and biceps forward are all being maintained throughout the activity.

Moving your arm to reach for the item in the cabinet in a natural angle slightly out to the side of the core instead of straight in front. Consider storing most used items within a height of your core to keep safer reaching heights, especially if the items are heavier.

Plan the lift, keep your feet base wide, load close, move your feet to keep load moving quickly to the destination while keeping your core still.

Practice using your arm with door opening while protecting your shoulder and spine by keeping your upper arm at the side of your core, which stabilizes the spine, and adds support for the arm. Then keeping biceps facing forward, use the rotation of your forearm, bending of the wrist and hand to operate the door handle. Open the door by using the entire body weight as you move your feet forward through the opening.

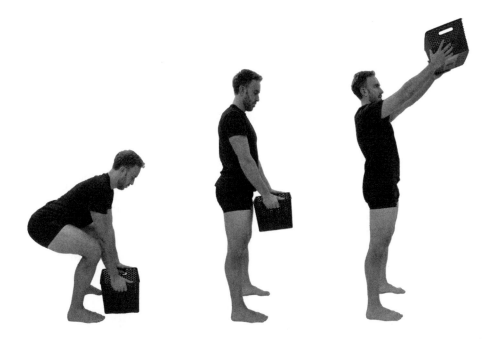

Reaching forward, keeping your biceps facing forward maintains best shoulder alignment. Recognize that the forearm turns independent of the shoulder, and in fact with better force and ability when the shoulder stays still as a base of support. Try opening a door and see how you begin moving your arm forward. Do you use your shoulder or hand?

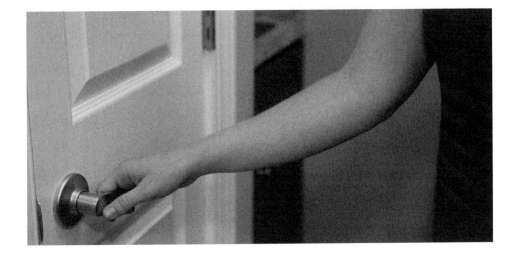

## 4. Stairs

Practicing each component of going up and down stairs in front of a mirror with a sturdy support beside you will allow you to visually assess your ability to maintain appropriate alignment throughout each part. TIP: Staying slightly on your forefoot as you ascend will help the spring-like mechanism of the foot stay in a more appropriate position. Monitor your core to ensure no changes occur; confirm hip angle, keeping it wide enough to maintain alignment, hip hinge forward slightly as you push off the bottom foot by raising onto your forefoot. This push up from the bottom foot simultaneously with

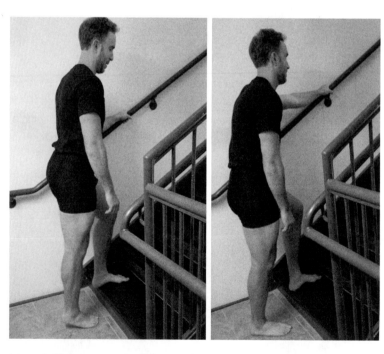

(above left) Correct: push off bottom foot plus top foot on ball of foot and hand on rail near side and hips hinges slightly forward.
(above right) Incorrect: flat feet hand far up rail and slouched core.

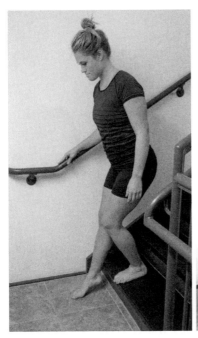 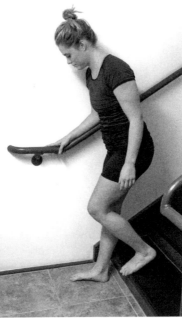

(above left) Correct: land on ball of foot on lower foot and top foot supporting the hips, bending as if you are starting to sit, hand on rail near side.

(above right) Incorrect: flat landing on the lower foot, feet turned out and slouched core.

pushing up with the forefoot on the upper step creates an efficient, safe, and balanced body use. The railing, if needed, could be held near the hip to push down for assistance.

Confirm the front pelvis bone does not drop when the foot lowers down. As a foot steps down, think about sitting down (avoid leaning forward) and land on your forefoot (not flat footed) and think about landing softly. If the railing is used, again, keep hand close to your hip to assist balanced body weight sharing.

## 5. Walking

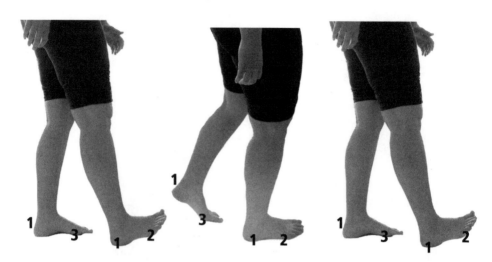

The goal is to reset appropriate sequence of movement with appropriate alignment for walking. This is a beginner drill. Start with one foot forward on your heel (#1) and front of the foot held up in alignment (#2 and #3) with back foot flat. Shift weight forward from heel to flat foot, while rolling onto the toes (#2 and #3) of the back foot. Arms should move with opposite leg. Then roll back to the original starting position. Repeat forward/backward heel/toe rolling drill in a one-per-second cycle for twenty repetitions without moving core.

## 6. Phone Usage

Take three seconds to use the equipment (chair) around you for support or have your upper arms at your sides for support. Bend your elbows enough to have the screen viewed in front of you while maintaining your ears-over-shoulder-tips position. With forward head position plus no arm support, there will be a consequential lack of circulation, no rest, resulting in overuse and pain.

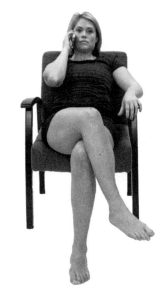

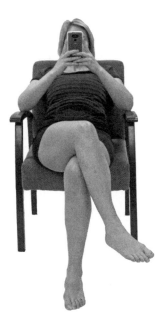

Using the "think in threes" tool to assess; left leg and left arm are supporting the body and the back is on the chair.

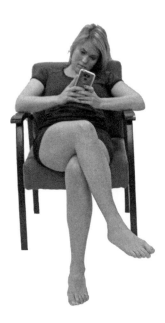

Legs, both arms, and back are supported on the chair with supported hands in front of face allowing appropriate neck position keeping ears over shoulders.

# Athletic Performance

Because of the competitive component of athletics, there is a necessary additional focus and more disciplined check in balancing the importance of the cost of competition with long-term body damage and potential risks. Obviously, there are many examples of life-changing financial consequences in the world of professional sport competition that present different circumstances for decision-making. However, the majority of the public, although often passionate, emotionally and financially vested, and socially dependent on their athletic endeavors, are not professional athletes. So, for this group, recognize your abilities and then understand that in order to perform at your optimal level you must allow the body to repair, recover, and rest. Listen to the language of your body, train in sport-specific, natural movement patterns and appropriate alignment and you will reach optimal performance for life.

**Patient Story:** *Jane Smith—I met Jane when she was a fourteen-year-old lacrosse player and had undergone knee surgery. She was struggling to return to sports and resolve her pain. After persistent conditioning, therapy applying the principles of the three steps, and lots of practice, she not only returned to playing lacrosse, but graduated from high school, and earned a position as a goalie on an Ivy League Division 1 team—a dream come true. During her sophomore year, she broke a bone in her foot and this ultimately required surgery. Loss of confidence* *and fear crept in. The workouts prescribed included strengthening her legs, arms, and core, along with cardio work, but did not include anything that matched what she would be doing as a goalie. When she returned to me in the summer, she had not played lacrosse in nine months. I attained a backstop, a goal, and had a kinesi-ologist, a former University of Maryland lacrosse player, working with me. Together, as a team, we helped restore Jane's mobility with appropriate alignment. By determin-ing where her adaptive movement pattern had been tak-ing her for so long after her injury and then practicing resetting to the optimal movement, she eliminated her fear and resolved her pain. She learned how to listen to and stay on top of her injury rather than let it run her life. She learned that soreness is normal when coming back from an injury and how to differentiate that from pain. She was able to return to her team in the fall cleared to play at one hundred percent. This was a month before her sur-geon said she would be able to start. By her fall tourna-ments in October, she was playing and practicing like she had never been injured.*

# Fitness for Life: Conditioning Guidelines

## Flexibility Guidelines

Flexibility is the amount of motion your joints can move or be moved. It is a measurement. Your flexibility is individual to you, allowing the mobility to perform activities. Generally, for life goals, arm and leg joints have equal flexibility. Stretching, on the other hand, is a tool to attain and/or maintain flexibility. Stretching exercises are necessary *only* if there is a flexibility deficit, and should not be confused with increasing muscle and related fascia and circulation for activity. Depending upon various diagnoses, such as Ehler Danlos Syndrome, extra stretching is often harmful. However, if you have degenerative joint issues, stretching would prove beneficial. Defining your specific issue with the assistance of a licensed professional and the application of the three-step method will allow you to know your limits. Go back and refer to the Geography of Your Structure and Alignment Checklist worksheets (pages 121 and 123) for check points. Be disciplined to not push through pain. When stretching, know the way to attain more range is active range of motion versus passive range of motion (someone pushing). When performing active range of motion, maintain appropriate alignment and hold for three to four repetitions.

Then increase range of motion each time, holding for two or three seconds. Active range of motion usually helps you gain more range of motion in the joint and has been found to increase muscular flexibility. Passive stretching (pushing) stretches the attachments of the fascia on the bone and can cause detachments and pain. If these sustained stretches are done (as in yoga) please know that you must wait thirty to forty minutes after these stretches before participating in activities such as fast running or jumping due to potential disruption of the tendon from the bone, because the muscle recruitment ability is essentially turned off. Static stretches should be performed at least an hour before an activity, but are most beneficial after activity and can be performed in the hour after.

You have the tools to make sure you perform any stretch correctly. The proper criteria is that you must be able to passively move your joint 20 percent farther than you would be while exerting force during an activity. Stretches, for effective release, do not have to be repeated more than two to three times daily if they are performed in the natural direction of your joint and in appropriate alignment, and held for thirty to ninety seconds. Use inhalation for three seconds then exhalation two to three times during this time period to enhance the release. Your muscles and fascia have no way to know if they are being released from a foam roller, rolling pin, massage therapist, shiatsu heated massage pillow or from you rubbing them. Trigger point dry needling (see Glossary, page 159) releases muscles more deeply and longer because needling is able to unwind the muscle spindles. All muscle release strategies, regardless of the name attached to them, serve as an opportunity to restore balance on all sides of the joints. Also, there is the opportunity to restore appropriate alignment, which is the key to strength. Stretching is a tool used to create appropriate motion to perform an activity. Off the field, if there is a need to reset movement, then stretching should be performed three to four times each day until you have even abilities on your right and left. Heating the area for ten minutes prior to a stretch will increase mobility of the tissue. A couple of the stretches you need to be wary of would be the hip flexor and knee to chest stretch. You will need to be able to find your natural hip angle. It is better to stay aligned versus pushing past your limits. Refer to the Flexibility Exercises in the appendices Toolbox on page 132.

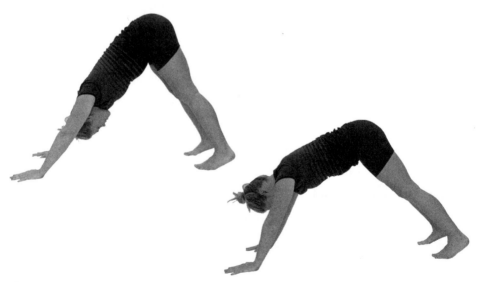

Left: Correctly sharing body support from feet through hips, spine then shoulders to hands neck/head aligned. Right: Incorrect load sharing and head and neck not in correct position.

**Patient Story:** *Allison C.—Allison had been struggling with EDS symptoms since she was ten years old. By the time she was eighteen, she didn't know how to manage her injuries or pain. She started eliminating basic activities that she had quickly categorized as "too risky" for someone with her condition. Her EDS had paralyzed her, and she had become victim to her diagnosis. Since she walked into my office almost three years ago, she's become stronger, more knowledgeable, and more active than she ever could imagine. She doesn't use EDS as an excuse anymore, but uses her condition as a challenge to help learn how to support herself. By resetting her posture and basic movements, she was able to almost eliminate her seemingly chronic pain. She claims that if she didn't learn how reset her body than she'd probably be lying in bed right now.*

## Strength Guidelines

Strength guidelines are another popular topic today, but are not the general focus of this book. However, I do have some reminders about strengthening. For example, isolated single muscle and core strengthening are not relevant to improving stability or protecting bodies from injury. Strengthening must be with alignment first in the same range of motion (natural), same speed, force, and endurance as your target activity. Combine patterns of movement as much as possible, and combine balance as much as possible, to build real-life application and

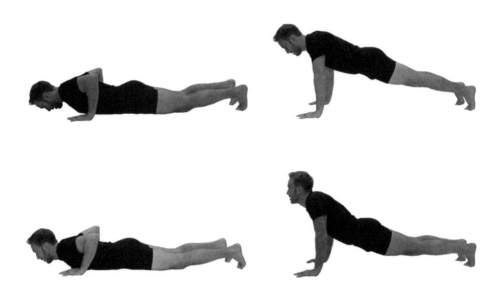

Push-up: Wrong start position—head facing up, not natural neck position; push-up start correct alignment feet to head/neck. At top of push-up correct: with arms straight, keep pushing core toward ceiling. Top of push up incorrect; neck position and no core final push.

adaptive reactions of your body. I have included references (page 156) with validated research for more strength guidelines. Remember the methods discussed in this book provide you with the freedom to enjoy participation in any type of strength program you are interested in.

The core counteracts the forces of the arms and legs, which provide movement and support for the whole body. Simply stated, the core is working to create a foundation from which the arms and legs move. The core is the base of support for the arms and legs. The spine bones are the actual core of support with the pelvis bones providing the attachment point

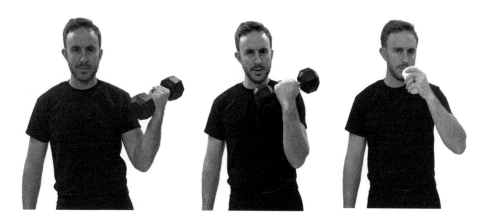

Left: natural direction of elbow curl; middle: traditional biceps curl; right: nature direction used in drinking.

for your legs, and the rib cage providing the track for the arms to move. In simple terms, stabilization is defined as unmoving or unchanging. During exercise, your core muscles are activated to make your pelvis bones, hips, and spine less likely to move. Where one's extremities create motion through space, the core acts to stop motion in order for the body to have a solid foundation to perform actions from a solid base. This is an important role the core plays when an athlete is performing any feat; i.e., sprinting, cycling, lifting, cutting, jumping, or any other movement. It is important to remember core stabilization is not about creating movement, but rather preventing excess and controlling movement.

Refer to the Strength Exercises on page 135.

**Patient Story:** *Brynn Hooper—Brynn came into my office with her throbbing foot, X-rays, and doctor's reports after being treated unsuccessfully for plantar fasciitis for over a year. She had been through months of physical therapy two to three days a week, multiple steroid injections, a cast, and finally was told her only option was surgery. So, she had decided she would just go on stretching and being in pain when she was referred to me. The first thing I asked her was, "What else have they looked at? Your foot is not your problem. If your foot were the problem, one of the above options would have helped. We need to look at your whole body." I assessed her posture, range of motion, etc., and found her alignment was not appropriate for healing or function. I taped her feet and explained body positioning and provided her with a few exercises and tips. In two sessions, she was feeling brand new. She went through the three-step method and learned a series of stretching movements, postures, and core activities. She has returned to running three to four days a week. She reports that whenever she feels an ache or a pain coming on, she pulls out her list of tips and tools and within a day she remembers why they are so important. She goes right back to feeling better and living an active, healthy life, pain free.*

# Balance Guidelines

Balance is the most difficult activity to perform. Balance exercises should be performed with rapid and precise muscle response. As long as gravity is a factor, as we all age it should be a priority to reset balance on a daily basis. Injury prevention is staying upright. We are all using balance throughout all our activities of life. For example, runners often blame core strength as a reason why a stride issue ensues, when actually, it is lack of control of hip motion in the air. Other people think their glutes are weak and that's why they can't get up from a chair. However, in my practice I found that more often than not the issue of poor balance begins with the feet and inability to control the actions both on and off the ground. That imbalance reduces the predictability of managing the body landing and pushing off step after step. Try the tightrope balance below. Also, this activity will help reset the entire body's response to ground and gravity. The tightrope balance activity starts with stationary positions and can be integrated to advanced movement patterns. In addition, Indo Board, other balance boards, and juggling can provide the neuromuscular balance needed.

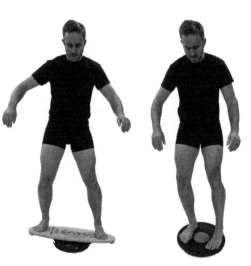

Balance Board is a great non-impact reset option for resetting hip control and sequence of foot to hip transfer of weight.

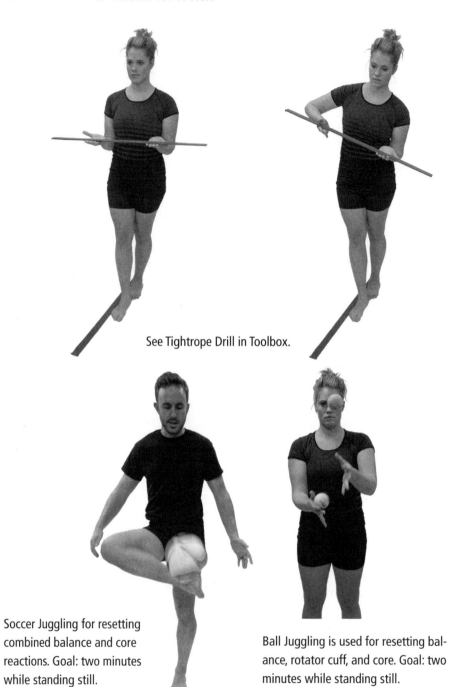

See Tightrope Drill in Toolbox.

Soccer Juggling for resetting combined balance and core reactions. Goal: two minutes while standing still.

Ball Juggling is used for resetting balance, rotator cuff, and core. Goal: two minutes while standing still.

## Foot Work: Move Your Feet

The twenty-six bones of the feet, along with the tissues and muscles supporting them, are responsible for the body's support and the transfer of fluids throughout the body. The systems involved are complicated and far beyond the scope of this book. However, restoring the most basic movements and resetting the balance of range of motion will affect all the systems of your body, and you may realize positive results. I have included some activities to try in the Toolbox (page 143) to improve the mobility of your feet.

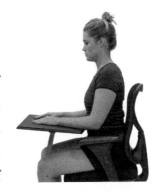

# Work Performance

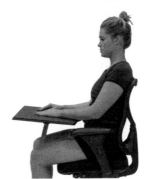

### 1. Stationary Work Positions

Confirming appropriate alignment, combined with modifying and adjusting the equipment you use to complete your job, can result in up to an 85 to 100 percent reduction in predictable work-related injuries, such as carpal tunnel syndrome and shoulder or neck syndromes.

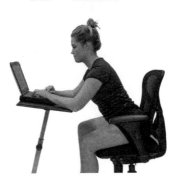

Top: Correct: Using wide base of support from feet to core, use chair back to increase core support, use arms on desk for better body support and allow muscles to rest while muscle are not used (choose to use your muscles, choose to rest throughout the day), allowing them to be used during later tasks.  Middle: Incorrect: Not using the back of the chair to add support. Unnecessary muscle work. Bottom: Alternate seated position from ground upward tripods of support. Thigh widths are wider as hip bending increases; supporting arms on entire forearm.

We humans perform most activities either supporting with, or moving from, our feet. Our feet are fabulous structures, containing twenty-six bones, and many muscles and ligaments, giving us a spring-like trampoline action. The foot uses specific muscles and ligaments to perform the proper propulsion, weight transfer, and shock absorption needed when taking a step. Proper foot movement is the first initiation of natural movement in sync with all extremities (legs and arms). Like the first domino pushed to make a row fall as expected, the bones of the feet are designed to be used in a certain order or kinetic chain for best effectiveness, efficiency, and safety. Best alignment with best movement sequence at each segment of the body starting at the foot allows the relatively unprotected knee joint (only three bones) to transfer the momentum and weight to the hips, then to a somewhat "stiff" core to the arms, where movement of one arm counteracts the movement and position of the opposite leg. Try this: Walk with the right arm moving at the same time as the right leg. This creates a stiff and unbalanced motion. Our center of mass (weight) is at the belly button, so to maintain an upright position as we move requires the principles of Newton's Third Law—for every action there is an equal and opposite reaction—in order for the body to keep going forward. Try it again and exaggerate the opposite arm-to-leg movement and notice the counterbalance effect that results. Without foot control, our structure is disabled, and potential for optimal performance is reduced. Perfection is not required, but resetting and restoring our feet to their full mobility is essential.

(right) Incorrect: There is no base of support from the feet, the core is not squared, the right arm is not supported on either the chair or desk, and the head is pushed forward of shoulder point.

(below, left) Incorrect: Feet are not supported in tripod of support, core is not squared, arms and forearms are not supported on desk, from the side no joint is aligned, and head is forward. Her computer is not positioned at eye level, and is too close to the edge due to the desk height being too low. Her right leg and wrists are the only thing supporting her from the ground up.

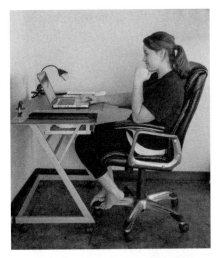

(below, right) Correct: Feet are firmly supported in the tripod of support, core is squared, entire forearms are supported on the desk, with height of desk allowing shoulder to ear height level to be relaxed, from the side everything is lined up: ankles, knees, hips, shoulders through ears, and finally upper and lower tripod of support are accomplished by adding support of body on front of desk.

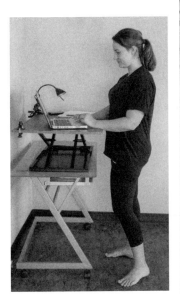

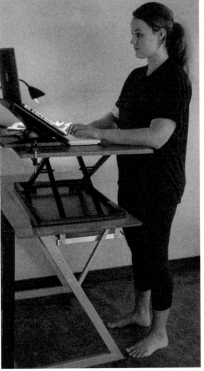

## 2. Manual Tasks

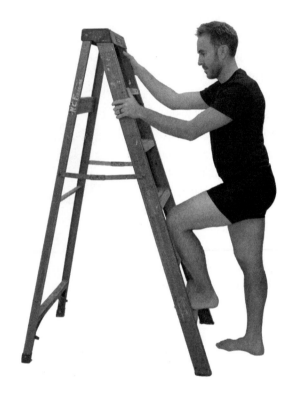

Pay attention to maintaining one arm support with opposite leg for best balance.

## 3. Driving

Thinking in threes, reset from your feet first, supporting your gas and braking foot in proper alignment and supporting the lower body in a tripod by placing the left foot on the dead pedal. Upper half of the body support must be found with alternating support side to side with the upper arms either at your sides and or with the arm supported on the center console or by adding a small pillow.

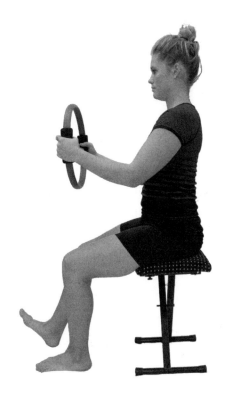

Change the angle of the seat every twenty minutes to maintain best spine health and circulation. The change does not need to be big. Preset positions can be changed at a light or when stopped in traffic. Hip health is especially enhanced with keeping the seat bottom lower in the front thereby keeping the angle of the hip more open. Remember to keep the thigh angle as wide as possible from the middle to keep circulation maximized.

# Keep Moving Your Feet for Life

## Predicting Body Breakdown

Ninety percent of all musculoskeletal pain issues occur as a result of overusing our joints, muscles, and other supporting structures, and shifting to a default movement or sequence, which is unsustainable over time. In the United States, it's estimated that 80 percent of the population will experience low back pain and 34 percent will experience upper extremity issues (Smartcare.com). It is estimated that it costs companies $80 billion dollars per year in workers' compensation and treatment of work-related injuries (Smartcare.com). This often goes on for years, unnoticed until the long-term effect of breakdown and damage becomes severe enough to make us pay attention and make a change. Compression on another part of the body, such as the ends of bones at a joint, secondary to adjusted mechanical effort or positions, such as slouching, poor alignment depressing the bone coverings and restricting fluid movement, or by the collection of waste products built up inside the muscle covering or fascia, causes a reduction in the speed and force with which the muscle can be recruited. The fluid movement eventually slows down and causes the muscles to react in a way they were not originally designed to, with altered mechanics, including limping or slouching. This survival process, if not noticed, stopped, or modified, results in an eventual breakdown of tissues, which occurs when damage happens at a faster rate than the speed the body can repair itself. This process is predictable and will cause pain, decrease function and performance, and can take years to surface. The effects will not be revealed to you by your brain until there is enough damage or performance issues to become an imminent danger and safety problem, such as falling.

Injury and pain are often separate events. To demonstrate this phenomenon, consider the times when you noticed a bruise on your arm or leg and cannot remember when or where you got it. Obviously, there was an injury to the skin with enough force to allow blood vessels in the area to break and cause discoloration. In fact, damage and injury most often occur in small increments without you being aware and without immediate pain. Go to the Compression Kills Worksheet on page 149 to experience the fantastic rapid interaction and adjustments the unconscious, Wizard of Bod part of your brain will make in response to changing demands on the structure with the fluid/nutrition systems and the muscles, when danger to one or all of the systems occurs. This understanding allows you to know how to use your conscious choice brain to recognize the language of your body and then reset it before there is damage or pain. Understanding the lessons learned from this exercise will help you appreciate the brilliant systems you have been given, and also begin to learn to read the language of your body to prevent future issues.

Pain, always "real," is in your head, adjusted by your

brain's response to input, prioritized by danger, altered by fear, medications, and understanding/misunderstanding of procedures and expectations, among other factors. That is why in the three-step method, the first essential step of rethinking is followed by recognizing the best plan to meet your goals, and must take into consideration the right, not necessarily the easiest, tools, skills, and solution team members. There is an imperative need to understand how the brain is able to function and help when eliminating the factors that diminish resetting potential.

The three-step method can be used to organize then solve health issues in the future. The method gives you an opportunity to make the right decisions and take the right actions, resulting in less pain, injury, and improved performance, potentially saving time and money.

## Shoulder/Arm Injury Prevention and Joint Preservation Tips

- Maintain biceps forward without leaning entirely on arm
- Keep all four quadrants of core still with shoulder tip under ears
- Arms should be either supported at sides if standing or, if seated, be open (naturally angled) away from core with entire forearm supported, elbow to wrist.
- Avoid sharp edges when working on keyboard
- Every 20 minutes, stop and shake arms/hands at your sides to rehydrate for 20 seconds; every 2 hours take a 2-minute micro stretch break to provide your muscles and tissues a mandatory relax/recovery cycle.

Alternate arm side use when possible; for example, switch hands when using a mouse. This allows muscle and circulatory recovery time.

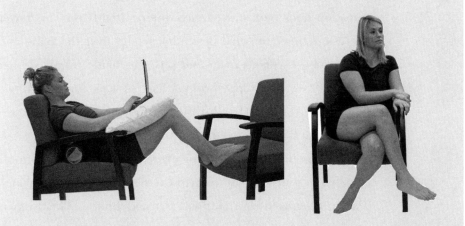

Left: An example of appropriate alignment that follows all the rules of "think in threes" assessment for working positions. Right: The most common adjusted positions restricting circulation, causing compression in joints, and eventual pain/breakdowns.

# The Full Body Example:
# Applying the Three-Step Method

Beth is forty-five years old and has two children, eighteen and twenty years old. She arrived at my office reporting right leg "sciatica" over the last two months, and low back pain before, intermittently for "years," that had not responded to any other treatment and was restricting her from everything other than work. Her injury history started with a fall when she was eighteen years old when a horse she was riding suddenly stopped before a jump, throwing her to the ground. No big or serious injury occurred at that time, but X-rays were taken and some low back pain started then, intermittently returning over the years. She competed in hunter classes over the years and understood excellent form and postures while riding. As her children grew, she stopped riding, had less time for herself, two children to care for (I call it the "30-pound child syndrome": one on one hip; another being pulled by the hand for a few years). She began running for exercise, because it was most convenient, but was not an avid exerciser and soon developed plantar fasciitis in her right foot. Her podiatrist told her to wear an insert and change her shoes out more often. She had chiropractic corrections when she would have episodes of back pain which would give her temporary relief. Time and life went on, her physical activities continued to decrease, life had become centered around getting through the day, including working at a pub a couple days a week. She decided to lose weight and started a "beach body boot camp" program. That's when she began noticing increasing right low back and shoulder pain. Both restricted her standing and movement tolerance to the point where she had to stop her class. When she arrived at my office, she had self-limited to the point she only could imagine a goal of pain management because of failed treatments and the level of pain and restrictions in life activities she had been experiencing.

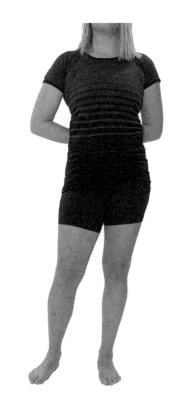

This demonstrates Beth's habitual standing pattern.

The following outlines how applying the three-step method to Beth worked:

## Step One: Rethink

**Define and Confirm Issues:** Beth had no medical reason/symptoms to need further diagnostics (skin color change, bowel or bladder change, muscle strength or numbness issue). Her issues were:

1. Constant right leg pain, especially in standing during her barkeep job within ten minutes and worsening throughout the four hours she works.
2. Both shoulders and neck tight, restricting her reach to highest shelf at work.
3. Unable to work out because of increased pain during and after boot camp workouts, not resolved with any treatment.

(See Beth's Activity Goal Sheet on page 151.)

**Solution Team Members:** Beth had no long-term help from any previous treatment or exercise approach she had tried; in fact, her symptoms got worse! We reviewed her current solution team and goal and reestablished a new goal list specific to work and daily activities instead of pain so we could measure results, and discussed weight-loss ideas with referrals made for a new solution team member option.

# Step 2: Recognize:

## Create a Baseline:

I assessed Beth's ability to attain and maintain appropriate joint alignment using the "think in threes" tool (see her results on page 155) in relationship to her goal activities and positions for work and daily activities. During her history interview and assessment, it quickly became clear that she was habitually maintaining her right foot rotated out to the right. She was able to move the foot to the correct position with coaching, but when not looking at it, the foot would drift back to the previous position and the arch of the foot would drop. This is the primary position, when maintained, that will eventually cause too much stress on the attachment of the thick supportive tissues of the bottom of the foot (plantar fascia). This position also over stretches the muscles overlaying this area, and shuts down their ability to be recruited to help support the foot, and to help lift the foot from the ground. This is consequential as the foot pushes off from the heel to the big toe. In other words, this foot position is disastrous to the chain reaction from the foot to the hip then through the core attachments on the spine to move her forward. While she had been sitting talking with me, she never once supported herself by having both feet on the ground. In fact, she never had her left foot on the ground at all, which is a very common habitual adaptation in people who experience this combination of plantar fasciitis, knee, hip, and back pain.

Try this: To see the dramatic effect support versus no support can have on your body, sit on the edge of a chair and cross your legs in a comfortable position, familiar to you. Feel how the foot on the ground gives some support for the core. Now lift that foot off the floor and hold it off the floor for 3 to 4 seconds. Quite a challenge! Now place both feet back onto the floor chair width apart. Best position with shared weight control.

Beth's right hip, low back, and left knee had been forced to counter the rotation of her foot both when resting on the ground and when she stood and started to walk. The culmination of sitting unsupported, slouching with a dropped forward right shoulder and a crossed leg, caused the muscles of the spine, which are connected to the pelvis then to the hip and to legs, to be affected by the sustained adapted positions, and subsequently the sequences of movements, as she demonstrated during her assessment of activities. The exception was when I assessed her horse riding position, which was appropriate. She also realized that she was able to hold that position very easily and without pain. Interestingly, she said she never thought she would be able to ride again because she was experiencing too much pain, but she wanted to.

**Revise Goals and Solution Team Members:** the only revision was to add horseback riding as part of her general fitness program for a balance and core strength component as this develops.

**Develop a plan to reach goals:**

1. For the purpose of this book, alignment reset was prioritized and should be from the feet up. Beth's primary issue in her legs that needed to be reset was the outward rotated right foot in combination with her habit of failing to support her lower half of her body in a tripod.

2. Instruction in self-care to enhance healing to repair the tissues.

3. Alignment reset of the shoulder practice.

4. Work task modification to allow her to use her body with appropriate alignment.

5. Return to general fitness with intentional appropriate alignment during activities being instructed during classes. Added two times per week the option for horse-back riding for core and balance components, but recognize that she needs to recover from her barkeep job, which is generally three days in a row, and not perform her fitness program on the same days.

# Step 3: Reset

## Implement the Plan

1. Beth reset by moving her feet to confirm that her mid-dle toe was aligned under her ankle crease then middle knee cap. Both feet were supported on the ground. The third point of support could be found either by using the arms of a chair, back of a chair to support her back, or by leaning against a wall to add support to allow her foot, knee, hip, and back adequate circulation to heal, and also have the best possible support and mechanical advantage for the remainder of the body.

2. She also was instructed in self-releases of muscles in her thigh with use of a rolling pin to enhance toxin removal and nutrient renewal, and use of heat two to three times per day for ten-minute sessions, especially before bed (a good time to allow repair).

3. Her shoulder issues were addressed with instruction in appropriate alignment using the ears-over-shoulder-point reminder, and she was instructed to have her colleague at work to use the trigger "think in threes" to remind her to reset her shoulder position.

4. Support modification, especially when working on her computer, but particularly when reaching for supplies and while prepping for her pub job. Practicing options and considering ways she could remember to change the equipment and tools she uses to work for her, not expect the setup to change for her. This means she recognized she could cut up her limes and lemons on a higher surface, allowing her to protect her low back versus her previous habit of leaning over a low surface to perform the same job.

5. We also adjusted and practiced using her body more appropriately for stairs and driving to stay supported throughout the time she completed these tasks. She learned an important lesson. Appropriate alignment allows most people to realize they have more activities they *can* do then cannot. She will return to fitness, including horseback riding, depending on how she recovers and reacts to these activities, as she resets upon reaching and maintaining her goal level of activities.

Reassessment of abilities is used to determine progress toward goals or effectiveness of interventions.

# The Other Rs:
# Recover, Rest, and Readiness

*Recovery*: defined as a time period allowing repair of tissue by having an exchange of fluids and gases to remove waste (toxins) and bring in healing restorative nutrients. The best rule to follow is when challenging and using the muscular skeletal system of the body for any sustained activity, statically or dynamically, you should expect that you should be returned to feeling back to your pre-activity rest state in about the same time period as it took to perform the activity. Common sense should rule. Expect with competition that damage or injury may occur from pushing to the edge of ability, which means that ability to maintain form and alignment appropriately throughout the entire activity probably will not be possible for several reasons. First, you might be in a contact sport, so this is an unrealistic expectation. Second, if you are a beginner, there is a high likelihood that you will be injured because you and/or others you are competing with or against are not skilled performing the activity, so either slow down, or practice, if possible, outside the competitive arena to avoid injury. Third, there are many environmental and other factors out of your control, including weather, referees, and equipment which contribute to increased injury risks.

*Rest* periods and sleep are used as specific restorative oppor-
tunities and should be considered strategic. Choose to use your
muscles to allow regeneration of fuel resources throughout the
day, choose to rest at intervals when muscles are not needed.
Rest for stationary tasks is movement and should be included
for as little as twenty seconds every twenty minutes. Rest for
active tasks or jobs is stopping and intentionally supporting
the structure of your body. Use the tool "thinking in threes" to
support yourself in tripods, with bottom half under the top half
of your body. This position is a perfect way to provide rest and
recovery throughout the day. It is effective using ten-minute
increments. Add heat to this position to increase circulation,
remove toxins, and increase nutrient supply for repair whenever possible throughout the day. Using heat then releasing
muscles and fascia surrounding them after you have finished

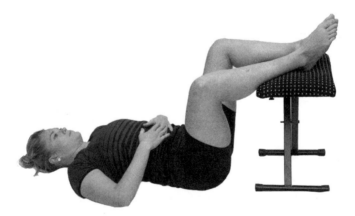

Recovery and rest: Seek gravity-eliminated and supported positions intermittently throughout
the day to allow restoration of circulation and repair. Hips and knees supported at 90 degrees
with feet together and knees apart. Stay in this position at least 10 minutes and consider using
heat to enhance nutrient hydration resupply.

most of the physical activities of the day is a great way to provide an opportunity for the body to have optimal rest. Adding
attention to using the "think in threes" tool when positioning
for sleep is the right decision to provide the best alignment and
support.

*Readiness* is the R to remember to check to prepare the body
for active motion, especially after being stationary. Natural
movements in the direction, speed, and ranges you need in the
joints you expect to use are essential for optimal performance.
This book is not intended to be a guide for this readiness but
understand that sitting still, even in appropriate alignment,
will compress the structures of the body, slowing the reaction
abilities of muscles and senses necessary for optimal performance. Work with your health professional to determine the
most important joints to get ready for your activity.

Below are general guidelines for everyday activities to
ensure minimal readiness and maximal recovery. For walking,
running, or any kind of activity, complete four to five repetitions of the hip rotation drill and shoulder blade and arm rotation drill to rehydrate the hip and shoulder/rib and arm joints
and wake up the muscles in a natural movement pattern that
you use in most activities throughout a day. As little as two
minutes will both help you recover the optimal circulation to
enhance repair and ready the myofascial system to allow
appropriate motion to perform the goal activity optimally.

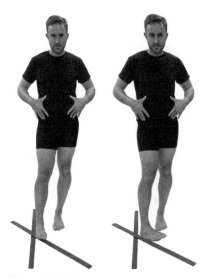

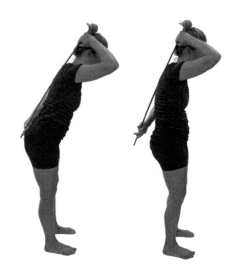

## Full Leg Rotation

Beginning with one foot forward with the outside of the foot perpendicular to the ground (#1 and #2) while monitoring front pelvis bones to bottom of rib cage. Rotate entire leg, knee, and foot inward motion of the knee cap on heel while maintaining still core. Goal: Rotate inward motion of the kneecap to about 45 degrees, repeat and check that each side has even ability.

## Forward Bending

Check to see if you can bend forward while keeping the core still. Bend only at the hip joints. Confirm with belly button to breast bone method, or using the stick on the back.

## Quarter Squat

Right: Resisted one-quarter squat, start position; Middle: one-quarter squat end position. Goal: maintain alignment plus speed one repetition/second, 20 repetitions. Confirm hip and core position.

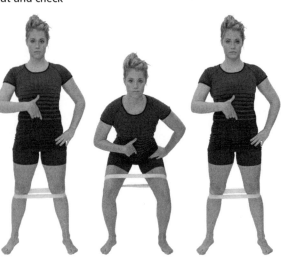

## Arms and Neck Flexibility Check

Check to see if you have even range of motion on both sides. Repeat 4–5 repetitions to warm up the body and also to recover from activities.

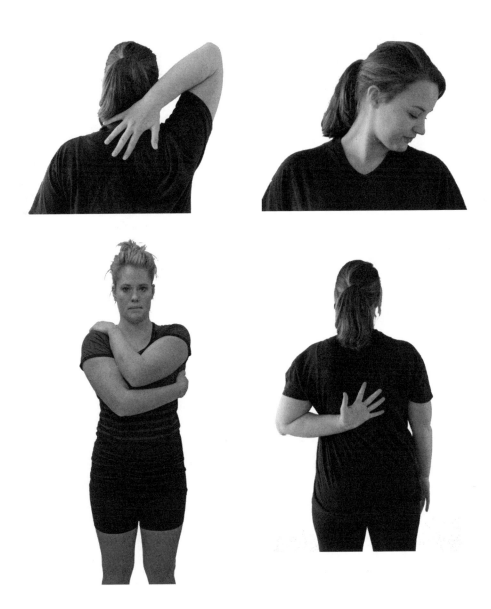

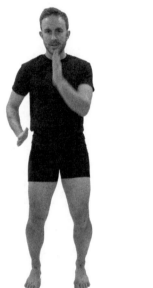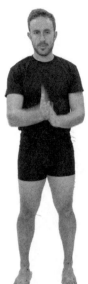

Practice reset arm movement sequence for running: clapping hands together in center of core.
Right: clapped hands moving apart: shoulders level/movement from shoulder then elbows then
shoulder blades

## Foam rolling

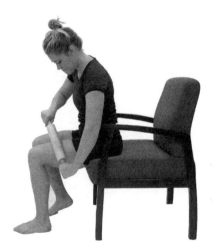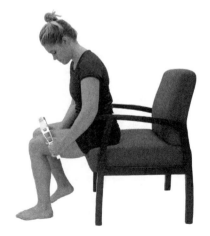

Use any type of roller, foam roller, even just a rolling pin, or the R8 device, both pictured on the facing page. Whatever the technique or device you use in rolling, take care to learn the proper use and avoid excessive force over nerves, bone, or tendons to avoid compressive injuries. Keep in mind, the relief that is felt is often because the signals from the nerves are disabled from the compressive force of the technique or device. Carefully check motion abilities first and then assess results after to determine effectiveness using the activities described on pages 112–113 as indicated related to your restrictions. Applying heat prior to these techniques will enhance results.

**Patient Story:** *Donna Lucente Surber—I met Donna about fourteen years ago when she began treatment to address significant low back pain and associated radicular pain secondary to spondylolisthesis (see Glossary, p. 159). The condition progressed over time and required fusion of L4, L5, and S1; however, she was able to defer the surgery for ten years by making significant lifestyle changes. These included regular strengthening exercises, correct stretching, and modifications to typical movement patterns that would often cause her to "reinjure" herself. Some of the changes involved altering the following:*

- Getting in and out of her car and bed
- Sleep positions
- Use of footrest and correct chair for various tasks
- Proper ways to bend, lift, and reach in both yard work and household tasks

- Taking frequent movement breaks when seated (every 20 to 30 minutes)
- Decompressing her spine through correct stretching and breathing
- Altering her standing posture to stop the collapsing of one side of her body when she would lean or weight shift more on one foot
- Relearning how to alter her posture to avoid twisting

These changes in her lifestyle have improved her overall quality of life and she has been able to sustain the changes in her body's alignment and prevent further deterioration.

# When to Seek Help?

Eight-five to ninety-five percent of all pain issues associated with muscle and bone fall into a category of "non-specific" cause, meaning they happen from a series of little injuries that are never really resolved over many years and the consequences finally build to a non-sustainable level, as opposed to one big injury or disease event. Obviously, the other fifteen percent are from a wide variety of issues, in fact up to 500 diagnoses. So, how do you know when to get help and who to go to if you do not improve when you have a pain issue? Remember the first sense you have: common sense. Rethink: Review carefully the three systems of your body and consider if there have been new changes in any of them for no apparent reason. Recognize: What have you tried to do to remedy the issue, how has it worked, and who you have used. (Reference the Solution Team Member Checklist.) Red flags are when you have been receiving treatments from a health practitioner or going to an exercise instructor and there is no improvement, the symptoms return immediately, or the same treatments are repeated with no plan to end or advance. Seek a diagnosis if you have sensation change in an area, change in bowel or bladder function, skin color change, and/or muscle use change; for example, you cannot lift the front of your foot, or you have difficulty holding your water bottle, or a new change in vision or hearing. Do not let fear of what the diagnosis "could be" stop you from seeking a diagnosis. You are in control of your own body and can give permission for procedures, but lose control of options if you ignore symptoms and miss a window of opportunity for healing because of fear. A consultation with your personal physician is a good place to start to rule out other diagnoses, such as kidney-related conditions, which can mimic low back pain, or certain lymphoma, which can mimic shoulder conditions, or heart issues, which can mimic a mid-back pain, to name a few. It is important to have the most accurate and expedient diagnosis to apply the most appropriate remedy for an optimal outcome. It is not a failure to need to go to the doctor or have a surgery if that is the only solution. Just use a method to ensure you are following proven solutions to reach your goals.

Use the tips, tools. and skills you have learned in the three-step method to ensure that you can reset and recover more quickly from whatever the issue might be. Remember, we each have been given an amazing body, designed for repair and regeneration, if we allow it, if we listen to our body, and take care of it for our lifetime.

# Summary

The three-step method teaches a systematic way to reset your body after adapting to default movement patterns that may have been causing pain, injury, and performance issues for years. The three-step method presents a solution that is tailored to your specific body's geography and structure and that allows you to intentionally reset the musculoskeletal structural system to become successful in the jobs and tasks you face every day. The primary challenge of this system is supporting a person within a position for an extended period of time or maintaining proper movement at multiple speeds, forces, and directions while walking, running, pushing, pulling, and/or lifting. *Aligned for Success* presents you with a new method to address the reality of what your body is telling you. Your body's language is used to assess where to start *rethinking* alignment issues, how to *recognize* positions and movement patterns and then develop and implement a plan to *reset* your body to attain your goals. Solving and removing previous default patterns or sequences of positioning your body between gravity and the surface you are on is a key factor to fastest and optimal results.

**Back Tips Injury Prevention**

- Move your feet and arms from the hip and shoulder sockets as you walk
- Always support your body in tripods from the ground upward
- Never slouch
- Change your position while seated or standing every twenty minutes

This book is about you taking time to stop and rethink the exact issues that have been keeping you from attaining and maintaining the ability to move through your life relatively pain and injury free, performing and participating at a level of your optimal potential. Balance the realities of facts, not beliefs, with goals for tomorrow and have a plan of action for today that is yours. Recognize how you are using your body then reset your body to reach your goals! Life is not a pain-free affair. Live it. The three-step method skills and tools will help you confidently move with less fear while regaining a future with more ability than disability. You can change your body to adapt and adjust to the environment and equipment necessary to complete activities that you want and need to do, which will prevent the most predictable injuries and performance problems. Reset your body from the ground up and you will be aligned for success.

# Appendices:
# Three-Step Method Toolbox

### Geography of Your Structure Worksheet_____Date_____

This worksheet is used to help you find your "geographical landmarks" so you are able to learn and repeat confirmation of alignment with confidence and competence.

You will need: a magic marker (or stickers); your hands; 1–2 full-length mirrors (flimsy home improvement store ones are fine and are usually under $10) so you can see front and sides; paint tape; someone to take your picture (that you trust to not upload ☺); and a yard/meter stick (found also at stores above) or furring strip.

Have someone take a picture of you from the front and the sides and print them. Then, as you find each landmark, place a checkmark in the box.

**Think in 3s:**

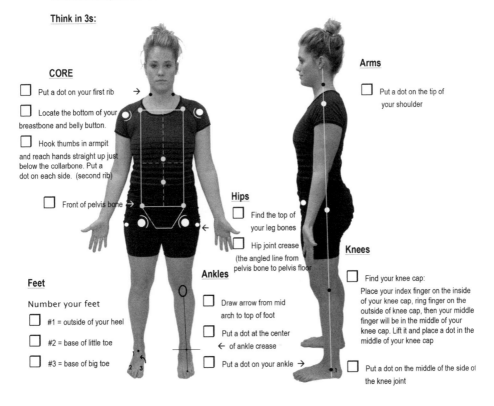

**CORE**

☐ Put a dot on your first rib →

☐ Locate the bottom of your breastbone and belly button.

☐ Hook thumbs in armpit and reach hands straight up just below the collarbone. Put a dot on each side. (second rib)

☐ Front of pelvis bone →

**Feet**

Number your feet

☐ #1 = outside of your heel

☐ #2 = base of little toe

☐ #3 = base of big toe

**Hips**

☐ Find the top of your leg bones

☐ Hip joint crease (the angled line from pelvis bone to pelvis floor

**Ankles**

☐ Draw arrow from mid arch to top of foot

☐ Put a dot at the center ← of ankle crease

☐ Put a dot on your ankle →

**Arms**

☐ Put a dot on the tip of your shoulder

**Knees**

☐ Find your knee cap: Place your index finger on the inside of your knee cap, ring finger on the outside of knee cap, then your middle finger will be in the middle of your knee cap. Lift it and place a dot in the middle of your knee cap

☐ Put a dot on the middle of the side of the knee joint

# Worksheet: It Is Muscle Memory?

Date: _____

**TRY THIS:** Place a piece of paper on a tabletop and a pen in the middle of the paper, splitting the paper into a right and left half. Place both your hands palm down on opposite sides of the pen. Have someone count down and then time (or record) how long it took for you to write your full name with your dominant hand from the time you pick up the pen to the time you finish writing, and place your pen back down on the paper with hands back in to the starting position. Repeat with the other hand and record your time.

Right time: _____ sec. Left time: _____ sec.

# Alignment Checklist

This checklist is a tool to recognize your abilities. Use every time you have a new goal to assess and need to know where to start, and what the most important issues are to reset your body to reach your goals. Assess if you can attain alignment positions in each part. Record with an "AA" in the Check & Comments section. If you cannot attain alignment, record an "NA," then record why you cannot in the comment section, including further information about what happens when you move, and if you are able to maintain these positions throughout the goal activity. Record plans for reset under "Reset Plan Focus." Reset your alignment abilities starting from your feet first using the information on this checklist for reset planning and monitoring. Confirm, reinforce, and become confident and competent with pictures or video to measure progress toward success.

| BODY SEGMENT | DESCRIPTION |
|---|---|
| LEGS: front feet/ankles/ knees (sitting) | Using three fingers on the kneecap, confirm that middle finger is aiming straight down to the mid-ankle and base of third toe. If not, move your forefoot, arrow at mid-foot, and/or knee position to align properly. Toes are flat and three points of foot have even pressure. |
| LEGS: front feet/ankles/ knees (standing) | Using three fingers on the kneecap, confirm that middle finger is aiming straight down to the mid-ankle and base of third toe. If not, move your forefoot, arrow at mid-foot, and/or knee position to align properly. Toes are flat and three points of foot have even pressure. |
| LEGS: side feet/ankles/ knees/hips (standing) | Knees straight: middle finger at side hip bone points straight down. |
| CORE: pelvis (sitting) | Seat bones even; right/left |
| CORE: pelvis (standing) | Front pelvis bones level; right/left |
| CORE: ribs/spine (moving) | 4 quadrants squared. No change in breastbone to belly-button distance. Notice which finger moves first to understand where to start resetting: top finger means start in arms or upper core; bottom means legs or lower core. |
| ARMS: hand/wrist | Middle finger "knuckle" aligned with mid-wrist and forearm. Notice which finger moves first in order to understand where to reset: top finger means start in arms or upper core; bottom means legs or lower core. |
| ARMS: elbow | No hyperextension, elbow and wrist bend aligned. |
| ARMS: shoulders | Biceps forward. |
| ARMS: shoulders | Shoulders level. |
| ARMS: shoulders | Shoulder tip below ear hole. |
| HEAD/NECK: upright (sitting or standing) | Thumb at ear opening, index finger at nose tip, level to floor (elbows out). |
| HEAD/NECK: | Even side to side and ears level R/L. |

| RIGHT | LEFT | CHECK & COMMENTS (pain, stiffness, unsure?) | RESET PLAN FOCUS |
|---|---|---|---|
|  |  |  |  |
|  |  |  |  |
|  |  |  |  |
|  |  |  |  |
|  |  |  |  |
|  |  |  |  |
|  |  |  |  |
|  |  |  |  |
|  |  |  |  |
|  |  |  |  |
|  |  |  |  |
|  |  |  |  |
|  |  |  |  |

# Activity Goal Sheet

*Please choose one number per activity for both the Pain Scale Score and PSAS Score:*

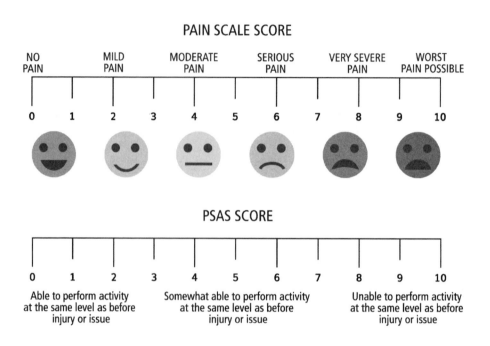

**PAIN SCALE SCORE**

| NO PAIN | MILD PAIN | MODERATE PAIN | SERIOUS PAIN | VERY SEVERE PAIN | WORST PAIN POSSIBLE |

0    1    2    3    4    5    6    7    8    9    10

**PSAS SCORE**

0    1    2    3    4    5    6    7    8    9    10

Able to perform activity at the same level as before injury or issue

Somewhat able to perform activity at the same level as before injury or issue

Unable to perform activity at the same level as before injury or issue

1. List the activity (i.e. walk, run, drive), then circle the appropriate category.

2. List how goal will be measured (i.e. 5,000 steps daily; run 1 mile in 12 min x 3/ per week, drive to/from work with 0/10 pain in 6 weeks).

3. List current ability to perform activities.

4. Fill in a score for both Patient Specific Activity Score (PSAS) and Pain Scale Score.

**Name:** _____**Date:** _____

**Activity 1**: (circle one): Work—Play/Athletic—Everyday movement (driving, dressing)

Activity:_____

_____

Goal:_____

_____

Ability Now:_____

_____

**Pain score:** _____ **PSAS score:** _____

**Activity 2**: (circle one): Work—Play/Athletic—Everyday movement (driving, dressing)

Activity:_____

_____

Goal:_____

_____

Ability Now:_____

_____

**Pain score:** _____ **PSAS score:** _____

**Activity 3**: (circle one): Work—Play/Athletic—Everyday movement (driving, dressing)

Activity:_____

_____

Goal:_____

_____

Ability Now:_____

_____

**Pain score:** _____ **PSAS score:** _____

# Solution Team 1 Worksheet

Name: _____     Date: _____

This assignment is to help you develop the best team to help you reach your goals. Research shows that when attempting to bring your issues under control it is beneficial for you to make your "team" as small as possible. Assess who is currently on your team, remove negativity, overlap of services, and underqualified and/or inappropriate professionals. Last, build a new team appropriate for you to help you reach your potential.

List all people who you currently consider part of your "team" (life). Do not forget perimeter friends, coworkers, family members who are trying to help, classes you go to, and the internet "sources" you have been using. Just list all of them. Rate if you feel they are a positive (+) or negative (–) on your team. Team 2 will be your new team developed over this program time.

## Physical: family, professionals, trainers, classes, others

| Name & credentials (licensed vs. certified) | Specific Role in Support | + or − |
|---|---|---|
| _____ | _____ | _____ |
| _____ | _____ | _____ |
| _____ | _____ | _____ |
| _____ | _____ | _____ |
| _____ | _____ | _____ |
| _____ | _____ | _____ |
| _____ | _____ | _____ |

## Nutrition: include internal medicine/general physicians, all "nutritionists," acupuncturists, and other sources.

| Name & credentials (licensed vs. certified) | Specific Role in Support | + or − |
| --- | --- | --- |
| | | |
| | | |
| | | |
| | | |
| | | |
| | | |
| | | |

## Summarize Changes and Actions Needed

| Name & credentials (licensed vs. certified) | Specific Role in Support/Goal Date |
| --- | --- |
| | |
| | |
| | |
| | |
| | |
| | |

## Notes

_____

_____

_____

# Solution Team 2  Worksheet

Name: _____          Date: _____

This is your solution team to achieve your best goals for life. Great job on examining your prior team, reorganizing your "toolbox," and developing a new one with the best team members for your goals and tools you can name and know when and how to use each! Use this format to regularly assess your "toolbox." As you grow and change, you need to use your new skill sets to determine if your solution team members are the most appropriate for your goals. Consistently using positivity, activity-based goals (function versus pain ratings), and current evidence-based solutions are the keys to success over time!

## Psychosocial: family, professionals, classes, others

| Name & credentials (licensed vs. certified) | Specific Role in Support | + or − |
|---|---|---|
| | | |
| | | |
| | | |
| | | |
| | | |
| | | |
| | | |

**Nutrition: include internal medicine/general physicians, all "nutritionists," acupuncturists, and other sources.**

| Name & credentials (licensed vs. certified) | Specific Role in Support | + or − |
| --- | --- | --- |
| | | |
| | | |
| | | |
| | | |
| | | |
| | | |

## Summarize Changes and Actions Needed

| Name & credentials (licensed vs. certified) | Specific Role in Support | + or − |
| --- | --- | --- |
| | | |
| | | |
| | | |
| | | |
| | | |
| | | |

## Notes

_____

_____

_____

# Flexibility Exercises

Goal: Even range of motion side to side, stretch fascia, decrease muscle activity. Repeat stretch 1–2 repetition, these can be performed up to 4X/day if you are attempting to increase mobility or shut down overactive muscles, at "bedtime" and within 60 min pre- and post-activity. Hold each stretch 30 seconds. NEVER increase pain.

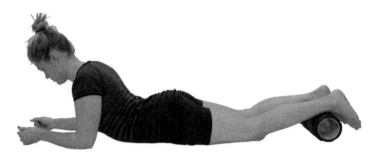

### Prone Prop

Lie on your stomach, legs about twelve to eighteen inches apart at your knees. Maintain roll under ankle creases or hold feet off end of bed. Keep front pelvis bones and the bottom of ribcage evenly on the floor. Inhale as you gently lift your breastbone off the floor as you prop on your elbows directly under your shoulders. Keep your shoulders-to-ears distance the same as when you are sitting or standing. Keep head relaxed. During the 2-min. session repeat 3 cycles of gentle 3 sec. inhale, hold for 3 sec. exhales. You may support chest with pillow or rest chin on stacked fists for more comfort. Goal: maintain for at least 2 minutes.

### Cross diagonal: Lats, lateral leg/hip

Thumbs toward the floor, elbows straight, keeping shoulder blades on the floor, bend knee and drop to the opposite side, then straighten letting leg drop, allowing the stretch from toes to hand of opposite arm release. Hold up to 30 sec. to 2 minutes. If held longer, perform up to 3 repetitions of 3 sec. of inhale, hold for 3 sec., then exhale within that time period for more comprehensive release throughout the core musculature. Goal: the straight leg drops to floor easily.

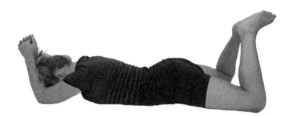

## Frogger

Bottom of feet together, thighs apart about 30 degrees, keeping core position aligned, elbows together in front, palms together, rest forehead on floor or arms, bring hands to head by bending elbows. Bend knees toward tailbone. Goal: touch heels to tailbone. Hold for 30 seconds or an on/off active release cycle for 4–5 reps.

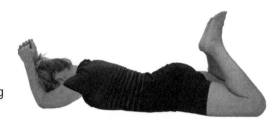

## Calves

The outside of the "back" leg should be perpendicular to the wall. Feel the stretch on the outside back of calf #1 and #2 of the foot on the ground. Maintain arch up and alignment of the foot and leg in all planes including knee. Goal: touch heels to tailbone. Hold for 30 sec. Or an on/off active release cycle for 4–5 reps.

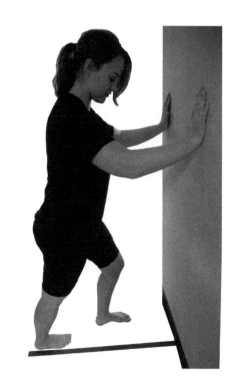

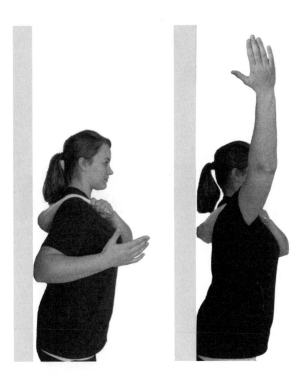

## W-V Ball on Wall

Place a tennis ball or spikey ball into a sock or newspaper bag. Position the ball on the most tender area on either side of the spine or muscle trigger point. Do NOT roll ball over bone. Bend your elbows to 90 degrees, with upper arms about 45 degrees away from sides, rotate the arm at the shoulder joint by reaching the thumb toward the wall. Hold this "W" position up to 30 sec. Move to the overhead "V" position gently by sliding thumbs up the wall while maintaining shoulder blades and ear-to-shoulder distance even side to side. Hold 30 sec. Return to starting "W" then repeat, in a 1–2 sec. lift to "V" then lower to "W" cycle active stretch, on and off for 4–5 repetitions.

# Strength Exercises

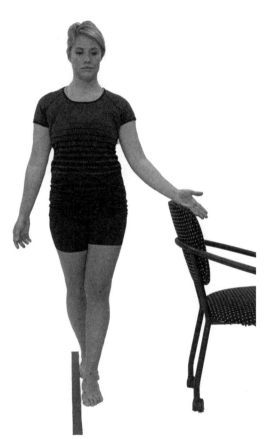

### Advanced Tightrope Challenge

While standing in tightrope alignment position, pull elbow toward side to recruit the latissimus dorsi (lat).

Turn the lat on and off in one sec. on then off pumping cycle for 20 reps with a force that will NOT allow a rolling chair to move on a hard surface while maintaining appropriate alignment in all body.

This drill resets the brain to learn an appropriate force and speed the lats need to be recruited to prevent you from falling over during standing and/or walking/running. Advance to performing this with your eyes closed.

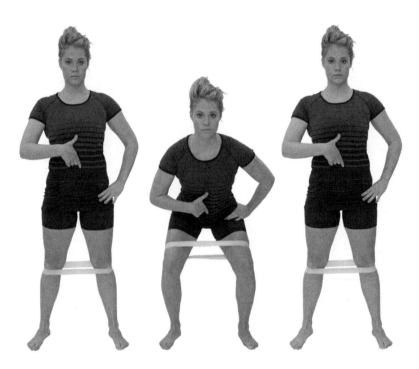

## Quarter Squat

Simultaneously push feet outward isometrically, maintain 1-2-3 points and pressure on band, either above or below knees. Maintain the belly-button-to-breastbone distance with hand as you squat. Goal: 3 sets of 10 repetitions in each repetition in 1 second's time, while maintaining core, leg, and arm alignment.

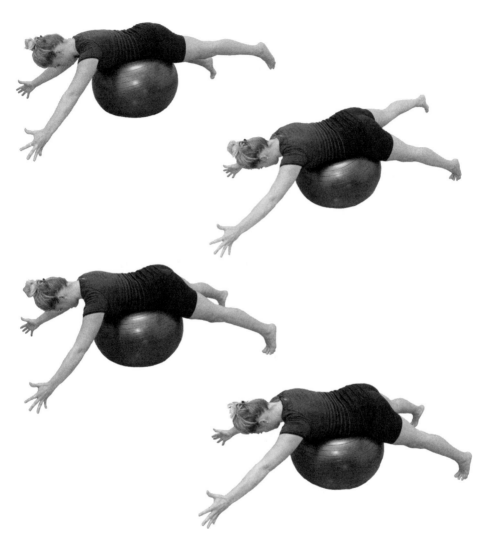

## Bird Dog on Ball

Instructions: Begin balancing on tips of toes and tips of fingers, thumbs facing up. Ball should not move. Lift each arm, elbow straight up and down, thumb up, and not changing support on other extremities. Lift each leg up and down, not changing support on other extremities. After 1 and 2 are completed: lift opposite arm/leg at the same time. Keep the ball still. Goal: 10 reps on each arm/leg in 20 seconds. Progress to 20 repetitions in 20 sec.

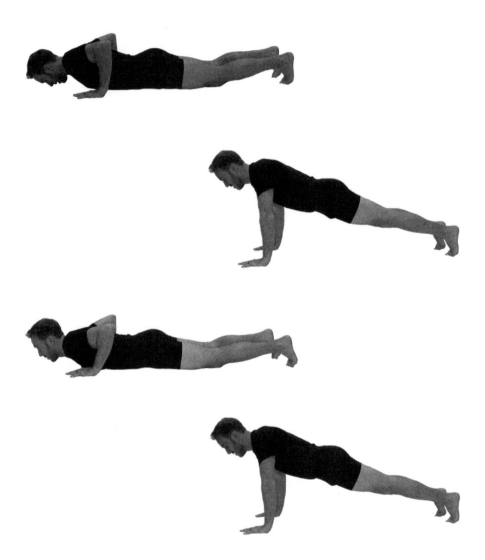

## Push-Up

The incorrect push-up position the head is facing up, and it's not a natural neck position, whereas the start position for the push-up is correct with alignment from the feet all the way to head/neck. At top of push-up arms are straight, keep pushing core toward ceiling. The incorrect top of push-up; neck position and no core final push.

# Tightrope Balance Exercise

This is an exercise designed to improve both sequence of your movement and also balance of your whole body. You will learn how your senses of touch, vision, ears, and joint position force muscles to counterreact and that this is the answer to overcome poor patterns of movement which cause pain and/or injury over time and will improve your performance and mobility. Here are the rules:

- Practice 1–2X every day until you can complete a level, then advance to the next level.
- Practice for no more than 2 minutes per session on a hard surface in bare feet with safety first: have a wall and/or other support handy to protect yourself from falling. Use a mirror and ONLY continue each session if you are performing perfectly. If you are practicing with mistakes, this is what you will be learning, which will result in predictable issues later on!
- You may split up activities of one foot versus the other foot at different times of the day if that is more convenient.

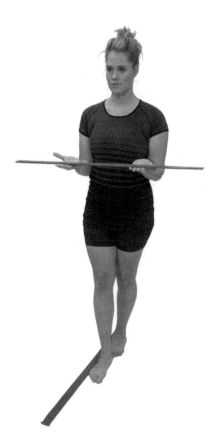

## Still Standing

- With outside of one foot and inside of the other foot on the edge of the tape, even forward-to-back-leg weight-bearing. Set back foot first.
- Elbows at sides at 90 degrees, palms up holding stick level.
- Core still (recruit about 25% max muscles): Correct slightly with the elbow toward the waist (activating the latissimus dorsi) to correct a fall on the OPPOSITE side of the side you are falling.
- Shoulders level and over your hips, under your ears.
- Visualize standing on a tightrope! Toes NOT curled.

Goal:

1. 60 sec. still each foot forward, eyes open, on hard surface.

2. 30 sec. still each foot forward, eyes closed, on hard surface.

3. 60 sec. still each foot forward, eyes open, on hard surface, head movement at a 1 time per second (see head movement chart).

4. Repeat above with arm movement and on a soft surface such as a yoga mat or Airex mat.

## Walking

- Same positioning as still standing, walking ON the tape forward then backward keeping a toe-to-heel and straight-foot step, making sure to keep mid knee cap to center ankle to third toe alignment intact. Move at a speed to allow perfect form and increase speed as you improve.

Goal:
2 minutes forward to backward walking on a 15–20-foot-long tape line at a speed of 1 step/second, keeping core still and legs neutral mechanics.

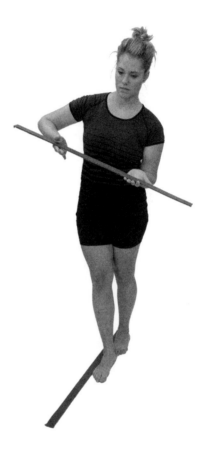

# Head Movement Chart

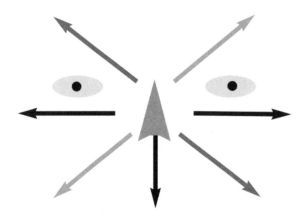

Stand still in front of the mirror, check neutral alignment with one foot in front of the other. Have a piece of paper ready to mark your results. One for RIGHT foot forward and another paper for LEFT foot forward. Then, move your head and eyes in each direction of the arrows, one direction at a time. Test how you are able to maintain your balance (and neutral positions of all body parts!). Mark on your paper with a green check mark on the arrow direction that you are able to move your head fully and return it to the starting position in 1 second and maintain your position and balance. If you cannot, then put the date you are testing yourself and a red check mark so you now know what you have to go back and work on.

When you finally are able to perform the direction of head movement, then write the date you have accomplished this. That will give you a record so in the future if you lose your balance abilities, you understand where you had the most difficulty restoring your balance to recover it again.

Goal: 60 seconds each foot in front, move head in all directions in speed of 1X/sec., 2–3X each way while maintaining positions of all body parts neutral.

# Footwork Exercises

## Readiness/Recovery

### Golf Ball Rolling

Seated, keeping knee-to-foot alignment, roll the golf ball under the mid foot 5 times in each of the following directions: Circle clockwise; circle counterclockwise; side to side; forward and back.

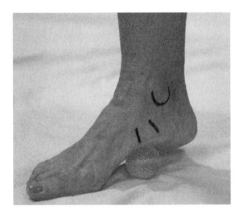

### Toe Bending and Straightening

Maintaining knee-to-ankle crease to third toe alignment, bend toes down then up. First individually, then as a group. The big toe should always be moved separately. Interlock fingers through your toes, or wrap your hand over the top of toes to bend down and hook hand under toes to stretch them upward. Take care to stretch the big toe slowly and not aggressively. Repeat 1 to 3 times for each toe in each direction, holding 15 to 30 seconds, then actively (by your own muscle power) bend and straighten your toes adding pointing your foot up and down 4 to 5 times.

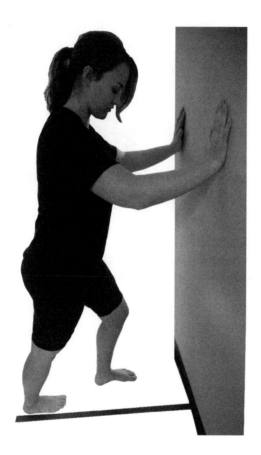

## Calf Stretch

The outside of the "back" leg should be perpendicular to the wall. Feel the stretch on the outside back of calf keeping arch up.

# Reset Strength and Movement Sequence

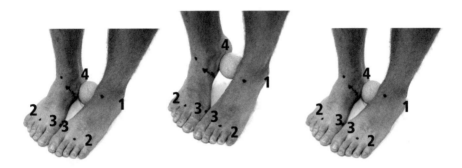

## Heel Raises with Ball

Maintain #2 and 3 touching in front of feet, arches up, ball held firmly. With no other body movement, raise heels from ground. Goal: 20 in 20 sec. Test: seated, with knees slightly less than 90 degrees first, advance to standing.

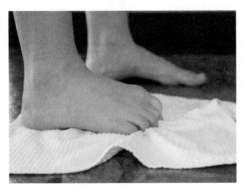 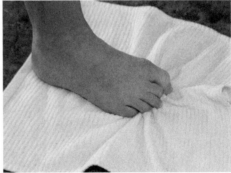

## Towel Scrunching:

Seated in appropriate alignment: 2-minute session, 1 to 2 times/day. Place heel at end of a hand towel and use the toes to pull the towel material toward you until the towel material is entirely "scrunched." Then try to straighten the towel again by keeping the heel down, now pushing the toes straight while pushing towel material away.

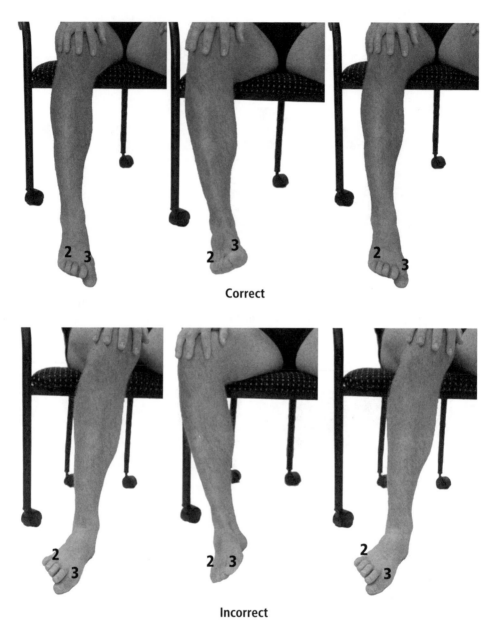

**Correct**

**Incorrect**

## Forefoot Seesaw

Goal: Seated then standing: 20 repetitions in 20 seconds, moving forefoot only. Advance each leg separately. When both legs are at goal ability, then advance to opposing direction each foot.

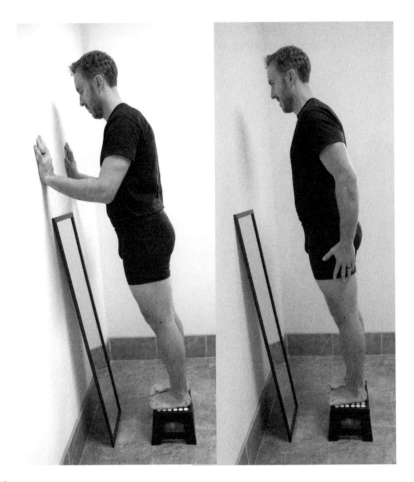

## Ski Jumper

Ski Jumper: Kinetic Chain (back side) test and training to reset: Ski Jumper starting position–
toes bent over front of step with legs about 4 inches apart and in appropriate alignment of all
3 structure parts. Hands on wall, mirror in front and to side to visually confirm alignment.
Angle forward about 15 degrees by bending at ankle creases. Tighten one segment of the
structure at a time starting at feet, calves, thighs, core, neck, then take your arms to your sides.
Goal: 10 repetitions: hold 10 sec., rest 10 seconds.

## Tightrope

See Tightrope Balance Exercise on p.139.

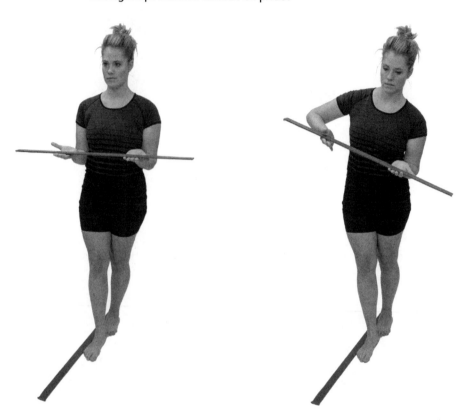

# Compression Kills Worksheet

Try this: bend both index fingers as hard as you can but keep your knuckle straight. Look at the top of the bent (middle joint) and notice how light in color it has gotten compared with the other part of your finger, but both fingers look about the same.

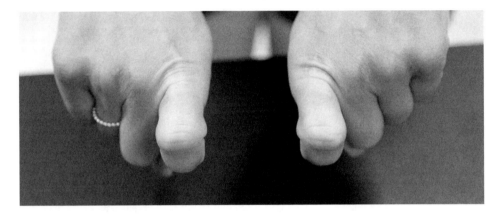

Now, push the bend onto the top of a hard surface (maybe 2 to 3 pounds of pressure…don't hurt yourself!) for 3 seconds.

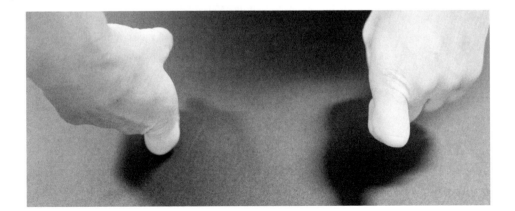

That hurt too didn't it? Your brain was getting an immediate warning from the bone ends that with compression (loss of circulation) there will be death of tissue if not resolved. Keep the other finger bent also. Keep both fingers bent for one minute and watch what happens to the area you pushed against the table top. Usually the response is an immediate "emergency" brain response to save the area by sending more blood and fluids to the area.

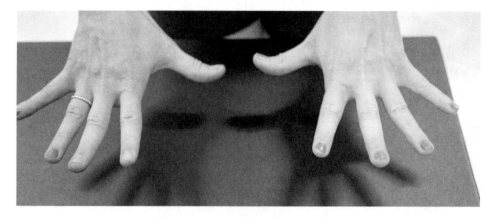

See the pressured area getting redder?

Now unbend both fingers. Observe how long the fingers take to get back to "normal." Also notice how your muscles feel that held your fingers bent for that long. Stiffness is the feeling from a combination of lack circulation in the bone ends and through the muscle themselves. More fatigued? Many people will notice overall swelling of the entire pressured finger. The average time it takes for the pressure spot to return to normal is 30 minutes for the 3 seconds of the 3 pounds of pressure.

This is why it's important to understand your body language to know when you are putting your body through unneeded compression, which in turn restricts blood flow. Compression kills!

# Beth's Activity Goal Sheet

**Name: Beth**                                    **Date: Today**

1. List the activity (i.e. walk, run, drive), then circle the appropriate category.
2. List how goal will be measured (i.e. 5,000 steps daily; run 1 mile in 12 min 3X/week, drive to/from work with 0/10 pain in 6 weeks).
3. List current ability to perform activities.
4. Fill in a score for both Patient Specific Activity Score (PSAS) and Pain.

**Activity 1**: Work

Activity: **Bartend**

Goal: **In 6 wks: Work 4 hrs, 3 days every wk. bartending/without pain or limited reach.**

Ability Now: **7–8/10 pain in right leg within 10 min. after standing at work in right leg and shoulder, not resolving for 2 days after working.**

**Pain score:** 7–8/10  /  **PSAS Score:** 5

**Activity 2**: Work

Activity: Overhead reaching and bar prepping

Goal: 30 min bar garnish prep and then bar overhead reach during the 4-hr service without neck/shoulder pain in 6 weeks.

Ability Now: Immediate increase pain with prep and reach limited by 40 percent or more.

**Pain score:** 5  /  **PSAS Score:** 4

**Activity 3**: Play/Athletic

Activity: Boot Camp Workout

Goal: Participate in 3X/week weight-loss focus and conditioning program in 8 weeks.

Ability Now: Unable to participate due to pain created from work.

**Pain score:** 7–8  /  **PSAS Score:** 10

# Beth's Alignment Checklist

This checklist is a tool to recognize your abilities. Use it every time you have a new goal, to assess where to start and what the most important issue is to reset your body to reach your goals. Assess if you can attain alignment positions in each part. Record with an "AA" in that section. If you cannot attain alignment, record an "NA," then record why you cannot in the Check & Comment section, including further information about what happens when you move, and if you are able to maintain these positions throughout the goal activity. Record plans for reset under "Reset Plan Focus." Reset your alignment abilities starting from your feet first using the information on this checklist for reset planning and monitoring. Confirm, reinforce, and become confident and competent with pictures or video to measure progress toward success.

| BODY SEGMENT | DESCRIPTION |
|---|---|
| LEGS: feet/ankle (sitting) | Middle finger on mid-kneecap, confirm alignment aiming at mid-ankle and base of 3rd toe? If not, lift arch of foot at arrow and/or move knee. |
| LEGS: feet/ankle (standing) | Middle finger on mid-kneecap, confirm alignment aiming at mid-ankle & base of 3rd toe? If not, lift arch of foot at arrow and/or move knee. |
| LEGS: knees (standing) | Knees straight: middle finger at side hip bone points straight down? |
| CORE: pelvis (sitting) | Seat bones even; R/L? |
| CORE: pelvis (standing) | Front pelvis bones level? |
| CORE: ribs/spine (moving) | 4 quadrants squared? No change in breastbone-to-belly-button distance. |
| ARMS: hand/wrist | Middle finger "knuckle" aligned with mid-wrist and forearm? |
| ARMS: elbow | No hyperextension, elbow and wrist bend aligned? |
| ARMS: shoulders | Biceps forward? |
| ARMS: shoulders | Shoulders level? |
| ARMS: shoulders | Shoulder tip below ear hole? |
| HEAD/NECK: upright (sitting or standing) | Thumb at ear opening, index finger at nose tip, level to floor? (elbows out). |
| HEAD/NECK: | Even side to side and ears level R/L? |

| RIGHT | LEFT | CHECK & COMMENTS (pain, stiffness, unsure?) | RESET PLAN FOCUS |
|---|---|---|---|
| AA | AA | Right foot kept drifting to the right and arched dropped. | T3 plus use K tape; modify seated positions. |
| AA | AA | Right foot kept drifting to the right and arch dropped. | Above plus add standing support T3. |
| AA | AA | The right knee hyperextended. | Consider hamstring and foot strengthening. |
| NA | AA | Kept drifting to the right seat bone. | Assess for manual therapy or cross diagonal stretch, T3 sitting. |
| NA | AA | Right pelvis bone higher. | See above. |
| NA | NA | Right upper quadrant higher than left and right quadrant bent forward. | K tape from top of right shoulder, diagonally down to mid-back toward left to remind brain to stop lifting shoulder. Lift breastbone and chest on right to correct quadrants to squared. Consider increasing attention to maintaining support of upper body by having arms on table/desktop when possible. |
| AA | AA | | |
| AA | AA | | |
| NA | AA | Right biceps rotates inward. | T3: with support and movement, intentionally have thumb of right arm pointing outward to position Biceps naturally forward T3: with support and movement, intentionally have thumb of right arm pointing outward to position biceps naturally forward. |
| NA | AA | Right shoulder high. | See above. |
| NA | AA | Right shoulder forward. | See above. |
| AA | AA | | |
| AA | AA | | |

# Sources

Aust J, Louw A. Pain is an alarm system—with brain education about how it is a positive as an "alarm" system. *Physiother.* 2005; 51(1):49–52.

Culler, AJ. *The First Book of Anatomy, Physiology and Hygiene of the Human Body.* Philadelphia, PA & London: J. B. Lippincott Company; 1904.

Duthey, B. *Priority Medicines for Europe and the World. "A Public Health Approach to Innovation."* [ebook] World Health Organization. 2013; 1–29. Available at: http://www.who.int/medicines/areas/priority_medicines/BP6_24LBP.pdf

George SZ, Bialosky JE, Fritz JM. Physical therapist management of a patient with acute low back pain and elevated fear-avoidance beliefs. *Phys Ther.* 2004; 84(6):538–549.

Greene DL, Appel AJ, Reinert SE, Palumbo MA. Lumbar disc herniation: evaluation of information on the internet. *Spine Phila Pa.* 2005; 1976: 30(7):826–829.

Hoffman MD, Shepanski MA, Mackenzie SP, Clifford PS. Experimentally induced pain perception is acutely reduced by aerobic exercise in people with chronic low back pain. *J Rehabil Res Dev.* 2005; 42(2):183–190.

Janal MN, Colt EW, Clark WC, Glusman M. Pain sensitivity, mood and plasma endocrine levels in man following long-distance running: effects of naloxone. *Pain.* May 1984;19(1):13–25.

Johnson, K. SAMHSA—Substance Abuse and Mental Health Services Administration; Oct 30, 2017. https://www.samhsa.gov/

Louw A, Butler DS. Chronic Pain. In: Brotzman SB, Manske R, eds. *Clinical Orthopaedic Rehabilitation*. 3rd Edition. Philadelphia, PA: Elsevier; 2011.

Louw A, Diener I, Puentedura E. Comparison of terminology in patient education booklets for lumbar surgery. *International Journal of Health Sciences*. 2014; 2(3):47.

Louw A, Flynn T, Puentedura, E. *Everyone Has Back Pain*: *Neuroscience Education for Patients with Back Pain*. Minnesota: International Spine and Pain Institute; 2015.

McGill, S. *Back Mechanic: The Secrets to a Healthy Spine Your Doctor Isn't Telling You*. Ontario: Backfitpro Inc.; 2015.

McGill, SM. Low back exercises: Evidence for improving exercise regimens, *Physical Therapy*. 1 July 1998; 78(7):754–765. https://doi.org/10.1093/ptj/78.7.754

McGill, S. *Low Back Disorders: Evidence-Based Prevention and Rehabilitation*. Ontario, Canada: Human Kinetics; 2012.

McGill, S. *Ultimate Back Fitness and Performance*. Canada: Wabuno Publishers, Backfitpro Inc; 2006.

Morr S, Shanti N, Carrer A, Kubeck J, Gerling MC. Quality of information concerning cervical disc herniation on the Internet. *Spine J*. 2010; 10(4):350–354.

National Institutes of Health (NIH). Available at: https://www.nih.gov/. Accessed 19 Dec. 2017.

Nijs J, Paul van Wilgen C, Van Oosterwijck J, van Ittersum M, Meeus M. How to explain central sensitization to patients with "unexplained" chronic musculoskeletal pain: practice guidelines. *Manual therapy*. Oct 2011;16(5):413–418.

Puentedura EJ, Diener I, Peoples RR. Preoperative therapeutic neuroscience education for lumbar radiculopathy: a single-case fMRI report. *Physiotherapy Theory and Practice*. 2015; 31(7):496–508.

Ramin, CJ. *Crooked*. New York: HarperCollins Publishers, 2017.

Ruschenberger, SW. *Elements of Anatomy and Physiology: Prepared for the Use of Schools and Colleges*. Philadelphia, PA: J. B. Lippincott & Co.; 1859.

Smith, TW. *Elementary Physiology and Hygiene: The Human Body and Its Health*. New York: Ivison, Blakeman, Taylor Company; 1884.

Vlaeyen JW, Linton SJ. Fear-avoidance and its consequences in chronic musculoskeletal pain: a state of the art. *Pain*. 2000; 85(3):317–332.

# Glossary of Terms

**Adaptation/Adjusted.** Synonym: compensation. When a sequence of muscle or joint use is changed from optimal use or from the original use for which the part was designed.

**Alignment.** Positions or state of adjustment of parts mechanically positioned to support and function together. Optimal, appropriate alignment (synonym: neutral) is when the end of one bone is parallel to the next allowing even weight bearing, fluid flow, and surrounding tissue tension. When maintained, this allows balanced muscular and other tissue tension and recruitment at still positions and throughout motion.

**Allopathic.** The branch of modern medicine, western medicine, using drugs or surgery to treat.

**Alternative Medicine.** Synonym: complementary; holistic medicine. Generally means treatment approaches of either licensed or unlicensed persons using non-pharmaceutical and non-surgical interventions. Can be scientifically proven or unproven. This term does not indicate one or the other validity level.

**Arthritis.** Painful inflammation and stiffness of the joints, most commonly osteoarthritis, is from lack of maintaining optimal, appropriate alignment. This compression then wear and tear on the joint surfaces over time causes destruction of the protective cartilage of the bone ends.

**Brain.** The primary organ of the nervous system. Comprised of soft nervous tissue contained in the skull of vertebrates, functions as the coordinating center of sensation and intellectual and nervous activity.

**Certification.** A process for recognition that an individual has met a certain set of criteria in knowledge or skills established by and for the purpose of a private organization for self-regulation, marketing, and an attempt at standardizing knowledge within that group. For example: yoga instructors, personal trainers, nutritionists, body workers, manual therapies, life coaches. There are often certifications attained or recommended by organizations for employment, and renewal of certifications is made mandatory by that private employer. However, there is no government oversight and no mechanism for penalty for not having a certification or renewal of a certification other than as determined privately with an individual. There is no legal government regulation or protection for the public if the person saying they are certified or advertising they are, is in fact, not certified. As opposed to licensure, which is mandatory for a practice of a profession, practice of a set of skills, and knowledge standardized by mandatory renewal of licensure. Penalties for failure to follow standards of performance and ethics are all are dictated by the state laws and regulated by a state licensure board for the protection of the public.

**CES.** Continuing Education System.

**Connective Tissue.** Tissue that connects, supports, binds, or separates other tissues or organs: loose connective tissue, adipose tissue, fibrous connective tissues, elastic connective tissues, cartilage, bone, and blood—binds structures together and forms a framework and support for organs and the body as a whole to store fat, transport substances, protect against disease, and help repair tissue damage.

**CPT.** Current Procedural Terminology: the codes used to describe a treatment for the purpose of insurance reimbursement.

**Credentials.** Aspects, characteristics, knowledge, education, licensures, certifications, training and/or skills, which are included in either being required by a profession for a person to perform a set of skills, licensure requirement, or are suggested or usually expected to be able to proficiently, effectively, and/or safely perform skills of a certain job or profession. General term for a list of some or all training a person performing a job or profession has completed but does not necessarily designate a level of overall competence of person listing the credentials.

**DC.** Doctor of Chiropractic. A licensed healthcare professional focused on the diagnosis and treatment of neuromuscular disorders, with an emphasis on treatment through manual adjustment and/or manipulation primarily of the spine seeking to reduce pain and improve the functionality of patients as well as to educate them on how they can account for their own health via exercise, ergonomics, and other therapies to treat back pain. They are licensed by each state after completion of a bachelor's degree, then a degree of Doctor of Chiropractic, including residency. The belief of the profession is that if the spine is aligned, the health of the whole body will be corrected or improved.

**Disc.** An additional layer of cartilage separating adjacent bones such as those found in between the bones of the spine called vertebrae and also between the joints of the head and jaw (temporomandibular joint, TMJ). Similar material in the knee is called meniscus.

**DO.** Doctor of Osteopathic Medicine. A licensed physician, often considered an alternative, holistic physician, able to practice in all fifty states, in all of the same types of specialties as MDs, including surgeries, and able to prescribe medications. DOs follow the same requirements to practice medicine and have the same specialty options as MDs for board certifications to prove advanced skill competency. There is little difference in the training criteria between MDs and DOs; however, the original foundational premises for DOs were different from MDs. The school for doctors of osteopathy originated in 1874 when Dr. Andrew Still, an MD, had recognized that the standard care protocols of medical care in the United States had drifted away from the understanding that humans are designed for self-healing and regeneration with optimal health. MDs of the day had begun nearly exclusively looking for disease and solving those issues with external remedies, particularly opium, alcohol, and surgical interventions. Dr. Still started an alternative medical training option, which taught to look at how the body could reach optimal health by restoring all systems. Until a few decades ago, mandatory training in osteopathic manipulation techniques, which allowed the physicians to enhance structural balance to help reset optimal health, was the key difference between MD and DO training.

**DPT.** Doctor of Physical Therapy. Physical therapists are movement experts who treat people of all ages and abilities, helping them improve and maintain function and quality of life. Physical therapists create individual treatment plans to match each person's goals, helping people improve their fitness and function, avoid surgery, recovery from surgery, reduce the use of opioids and other drugs, and partner in their own care. Physical therapists work in all fields of medical, school, military, industrial, and home settings. Physical therapists are trained to assess and treat the body as a whole integrated structure. All entry level physical therapists are licensed by a state governing board after completing an accredited mandated college curriculum that includes both comprehensive medical-based classroom coursework, including extensive anatomy, physiology, pathology, kinesiology, and specific internships. To maintain licensure to practice, a physical therapist must complete approved required educational courses every two years.

**Dry Needling.** Trigger point dry needling employs the use of a very small solid needle inserted into the muscle belly, which mechanically releases the excessive tension in the muscles.

**Dysfunction.** Abnormality or impairment or compensation in the function of a specified bodily organ/system.

**Eastern Medicine.** Encompasses many different practices, such as acupuncture (Chinese medicine), massage therapy, and any other approach currently in use in the world having originated in the eastern hemisphere and used to diagnose and/or treat and/or promote optimal health and well-being in humans. Included are yoga, many forms of meditation (now applying mindfulness), Reiki, many forms of movement to promote relaxation and calm, non-industrially produced food and medicinal products used particularly in Chinese medicine.

**EDS. Ehlers Danlos Syndrome.** A heritable disorder of connective tissue characterized by easy bruising, joint hypermobility, skin laxity, weakness of tissues; many different types.

**Energy.** General term used in the world of medicine and "healing" as a force or power. As a healer, a person has "good energy," a powerful personality, or unexplainable force. The human body has an electromagnetic field often referred to as "energy," and is mobilized, manipulated to enhance and change the functioning of the body with use of suggestion (mindfulness, intention), use of inserted needles (acupuncture and dry needling), and use of touch (Zero balancing), and many other examples. At this point in history, these techniques have a lot of overlap, and science has not fully proved all treatment protocols. This proof is further complicated by the fact that every person has their individual energy (electromagnetic) field, which affects every person they are near. Looking for "energy workers" with the most formal education that includes actual science including anatomy, physiology, and physics makes the most common sense for safety and effectiveness.

**Ergonomics.** Study of people's efficiency in their working environment, also called biotechnology; applied science concerned with designing and arranging equipment and tools that people use so that their interactions can be most efficient and safe. It does not indicate or imply teaching the operator use of or modification of equipment or their own bodies.

**Ergonomist.** An engineer that designs equipment for completion of work-specific tasks for the workplace, intended to maximize productivity and minimize the operator's injury risk, fatigue, and discomfort. The design criteria of the equipment such as chairs, grip sizes, desk and work heights generally are made for the average size of the population expected to be using that equipment. It does not indicate or inply teaching the operator how to use and or modify the equipment.

**Fitness.** A general term usually used to describe the state of a person's abilities to function in performing tasks of life including play, work, and daily activities. Components of fitness measured and addressed to attain and maintain optimal physical fitness should include: cardiovascular capacity, flexibility, strength, balance, agility, and mental focus relevant to an individual's activities.

**Fluid/Hydration Systems.** Components in the body responsible for transport and management of nutrients and waste materials in the body in a liquid form. Includes blood, lymph, cerebral spinal fluid, synovial fluid (lubricant in joint spaces).

**Health.** The dynamic state functioning of the body systems at any time. Optimal health is the very best the systems can operate to maintain the use of the body in all activities of life, including work, play and self-care, injury, and disease management

**Holistic.** Synonym: Comprehensive, entire. In medical or pseudo-medical (non-licensed) approaches, this is a way of looking at issues and solutions from a whole, comprehensive body perspective. Holistic considers not just the body, but all factors, including but not limited to social, environmental, mental, organic, inorganic, and not just one part of the body, but all different systems are taken into account. Not specific to "eastern" or "western" medical diagnostics and solutions planning and implementation, but an approach to these.

**Integrated.** Various parts or aspects linked or coordinated together, meshed together. Indicates corroboration of care and solutions implementation by more than one profession or person. There is no required level of corroboration and the word is used frequently as a marketing tool.

**Licensed.** A mandatory process determined and regulated by federal, state, and/or local government of attaining then maintaining permission to practice and promote that an individual can and is performing an occupation or profession as mandated and regulated by educational requirements and laws, standards with penalties for failure to comply. An individual must pass a licensing exam after mandatory/required uniform education in their field, then have continuing education on a regular basis, set by the law, to be able to continue practice. The public is protected by a set of rules and laws the practitioners must follow with required investigation. If questionable practices are reported to the board, then specific actions are taken to ensure safe practice to maintain licensure of the practitioners. Licenses must be displayed in the place of practice, and the public can contact a board of a profession to determine licensure status.

**MD.** Doctor of Medicine. A licensed physician able to practice in all fifty states, in all types of specialties, and who can prescribe medications, perform surgeries, and has options for specialized board

certifications to prove advanced skill competency. Often called
allopathic medical practitioners, MDs were first described in the
United States in 1810 by the founder of homeopathic medicine,
Samuel Hahnemann, to describe the practice of a physician who
used substances and/or approaches to treat the symptoms of a
disease, not the cause, versus Hahnemann's practice of seeking to
prevent illness or remove the cause of an illness. Currently, becoming an MD has the same requirements as a Doctor of Osteopathy
to attain and maintain licensure to practice.

**Meaningful Movement.** Natural movement that is relevant to activities of daily living in work, play, or self-care. Synonym: functional
movement.

**Meniscus.** A thin fibrous cartilage between the surfaces of some
joints; i.e., knee, facet joints, temporomandibular joints (TMJ),
designed for additional padding protection for the end of the
bones when the joints have multiple movement angles that can
occur. These joints move more than a forward-backward hinging
motion. They also glide and rotate. The shape of the menisci also
adds some stability to the joint when loaded with proper alignment.

**Mind.** The part of the brain that allows conscious choice and
decision-making. The part of the brain where you learn new information, that allows you to reset the way you respond to and
change behaviors and habits.

**Osteoarthritis.** "Wear-tear" arthritis, degenerative joint "disease,"
when the protective cartilage on the ends of bones wears down.
Causes can be a single incident, or minor repeated compression
of one bone end on the next bone end, pressing on each other
when not maintained in appropriate alignment over time.

**Out.** Terminology used to indicate the ends of bones are "out of alignment," meaning they are not parallel to each other, most often

due to muscular or other soft tissue imbalance.

**Performance.** The purposeful completion of a task. The task components can be measured.

**Position.** Description of one body segment in relationship to another segment or segments such as the foot in relationship to the shin and the shin in relationship to the thigh. Position can also be described as the relationship between the connections of one bone to the next, which are joints. For example, knee to ankle.

**Posture.** The summation of all body segments or parts being held in a position while still, such as in sitting or standing, or positions at any moment during movement. The word posture itself does not indicate good or bad, still or moving. There must be a qualifying indicator such as "appropriate" or "optimal," "functional," and further descriptors may be added to clarify the fact that a posture is a summation of the body parts in a moment in time, not one position all of the time.

**Proper Alignment.** The joints of the body each have bone ends parallel to each other to allow optimal circulation, support, muscular mechanically advantaged recruitment and movement and nervous system function. "Think in threes" is the tool used to confirm at any time if proper alignment is being attained and/or maintained.

**Rheumatoid.** Chronic inflammatory, autoimmune disorder diagnosed by a rheumatologist and a blood test. Rheumatoid arthritis affects the lining of your joints, causing painful swelling that can eventually result in bone erosion.

**Somatic.** Dealing with the body (separate from the brain, nervous system, mind/psyche).

**Spondylolisthesis.** A slip of one spine bone (vertebrae) on the other which may cause a pinch and malfunction of the nerves and muscles associated with them. Usually caused from a severe accidental hit or fall or repeated excessive forward or backward bending of the spine hinging at one level of the spine, finally often breaking the connecting bridges of the joints from one vertebrae to the next, allowing the slide.

**Sprain.** A tearing of the ligaments connecting one bone to the next. Graded as a grade 1, 2, or 3, with 3 being a complete tear. A sprain will disrupt the sensory feedback to the brain, potentially slowing down muscular responses to protect injury risk.

**Strain.** Term used to describe a non-tearing overstretching of any soft tissue of the body including fascia, muscle, capsule, ligament, tendons.

**Stretching.** Sustained pressure on any tissue exceeding normal length of a tissue. Sustained lengthening of tissue either intentional stretching (massage, foam roller, rolling pin, R8) or unintentional stretching such as slouching, staying in positions of poor alignment, the result is a decrease in the ability to use or recruit the use of a muscle for a period of time. If the ligament or tendon is stretched, the sensors that tell the brain information about tension on that structure are turned down or turned off for a period of time, causing a risk of injury if used improperly.

**Structures of the body.** Complex of anatomical parts that compose 1) support for the body: the skeleton: arms, legs, and core, spine bones; 2) containers for the nervous and fluid/gas systems: head, stomach, heart, lungs, intestines, and all other food and waste processing organs, blood and lymph vessels, craniosacral sac; and 3) transporters of information: brain, spinal cord, and nerves.

**Subluxation.** Partial dislocation.

**Syndrome.** A group of symptoms that consistently occurs together or a condition characterized by a set of associated symptoms.

**Tightness.** A sensation of lack of movement or feeling limited movement from a fullness in tissue.

**Wellness.** Synonyms: well-being, fitness. A state of being or pursuing optimal health and making choices dynamically in mental, physical, social, and environmental arenas. It is not simply absence of disease.

**Western Medicine.** Purely described, but no longer taught in schools in this manner: medical doctors, nurses, pharmacists treat symptoms with pharmaceuticals, use of technologies, and surgeries to diagnose and treat. Described as lacking consideration of other factors such as mind and spirit to diagnose and treat. This is versus the approach of "Eastern" medicine, which uses natural organic herbs, oils, and no technologies or surgeries to diagnose and treat.

# Acknowledgments

*Aligned for Success* was a team effort. The team captain and publisher David Wilk, with editor, Jeremy Townsend, endured my seemingly endless rewrites and babblings, and thankfully coached me to the finish line. Thank you for your professionalism, persistence, and patience, for which I will always be so grateful.

Many people were part of making this book a reality. From the initial idea to completion of the book, my son Tim and husband David served as sounding boards for ideas as well as valuable readers. Tim was working for my company at the time and was pivotal in bridging the age gap, providing relevance and reality checks, and in moving the project forward. What an amazing journey we have had, on and off the field! Thank you for all you continue to teach me.

Karri Ellen Johnson followed in Tim's footsteps. Our team solidified when Karri Ellen, Micaila Ryder, and Tim volunteered to be the models for the photographs. We had some very fun photo shoots in the competent hands of our graphics leader Kristen Sullivan. Kristen's talents as a photographer and her knowledge of graphics were invaluable.

Heather Macintosh, thank you for pulling the "Wizard" out of my head and onto paper!

I will never stop being in awe of and grateful to all of the brilliant and thoughtful clinicians and researchers who have been strong enough to challenge what is "known" and what is "true," then discovering how to apply these facts to help us all move forward. Specifically, I have been very influenced by Dr. Stuart McGill, Dr. Vladamir Janda, Dr. Phillip Greenman, and Richard Jackson, PT, OCS. Their humility about their impact on the field and their adherence to the principles of science are commendable. All four have set the groundwork for finding future optimal health solutions.

The principles and methods included in this book come from a lifetime of professional experience. The lessons I've learned from my patients were the building blocks to make this book possible. I am humbled by the faith that others have placed in me over the many years I have been a physical therapist and am truly grateful to each individual who has joined me in this journey. Without their trying and succeeding and sometimes failing but trying again, there would be no progress. Thank you!

To my friends, family, Rose Gibbs, and Betsy Meyer, who have all been involved with long discussions about how we can age the best and most appropriately, avoid injury, and make sense of the medical system today, I thank all of you for listening, challenging me, giving me new ideas, directions, picking me up, and pushing me forward.

To my readers, my goal in writing this book is to offer one piece of information that will enhance your health and help you reach your own potential.

# About the Author

Brenda Shaeffer, PT, DPT, has been a licensed physical therapist since 1978. She has a doctorate in physical therapy from Simmons College, a bachelor of science from Cleveland State University, and attended The Ohio State University and Mary Washington College. She has been a private practitioner since 1981, and has been an innovator in the field of physical therapy in business and treatment approaches in orthopedics and sports, treating athletes at every level. She is experienced in postsurgical rehab and neurologic disease care, including ALS.

Dr. Shaeffer has a long history of developing and implementing ergonomic solutions and work performance enhancement programs, work hardening and treatment with companies including Honda of America, General Motors, Nationwide Insurance, International Harvester, UPS, and Roadway among others.

Dr. Brenda Shaeffer's background as an elite athlete in gymnastics and acrosports and as a national sailboat racer and coach in both sports gives her an understanding of issues associated with recovering from injury and performing at the highest levels.

"I strive to help every patient help themselves to understand and reach their potential at any age and any stage of life."